The No S* Diet

The Strikingly Simple Weight-Loss Strategy
That Has Dieters Raving—and Dropping Pounds

The No S* Diet

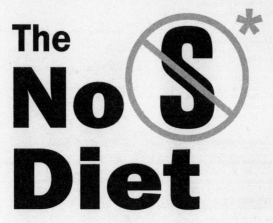

* No Snacks No Sweets No Seconds
Except on Days that Start with S

Reinhard Engels and Ben Kallen

A PERIGEE BOOK

A PERIGEE BOOK
Published by the Penguin Group
Penguin Group (USA) Inc.
375 Hudson Street, New York, New York 10014, USA
Penguin Group (Canada), 90 Eglinton Avenue East, Suite 700, Toronto, Ontario M4P 2Y3, Canada (a division of Pearson Penguin Canada Inc.)
Penguin Books Ltd., 80 Strand, London WC2R 0RL, England
Penguin Group Ireland, 25 St. Stephen's Green, Dublin 2, Ireland (a division of Penguin Books Ltd.)
Penguin Group (Australia), 250 Camberwell Road, Camberwell, Victoria 3124, Australia (a division of Pearson Australia Group Pty. Ltd.)
Penguin Books India Pvt. Ltd., 11 Community Centre, Panchsheel Park, New Delhi—110 017, India
Penguin Group (NZ), 67 Apollo Drive, Rosedale, North Shore 0632, New Zealand (a division of Pearson New Zealand Ltd.)
Penguin Books (South Africa) (Pty.) Ltd., 24 Sturdee Avenue, Rosebank, Johannesburg 2196, South Africa

Penguin Books Ltd., Registered Offices: 80 Strand, London WC2R 0RL, England

While the author has made every effort to provide accurate telephone numbers and Internet addresses at the time of publication, neither the publisher nor the author assumes any responsibility for errors, or for changes that occur after publication. Further, the publisher does not have any control over and does not assume any responsibility for author or third-party websites or their content.

First edition: March 2008

Library of Congress Cataloging-in-Publication Data

Engels, Reinhard.
   The no S diet : no snacks no sweets no seconds except on days that start with S / Reinhard Engels and Ben Kallen. — 1st ed.
      p. cm.
   "The strikingly simple weight-loss strategy that has dieters raving—and dropping pounds."
   ISBN 978-0-399-53404-1
   1. Reducing diets.   I. Kallen, Ben.   II. Title.
   RM222.2.E528 2008
   613.2'5—dc22   2007038930

PRINTED IN THE UNITED STATES OF AMERICA

10 9 8 7 6 5 4 3 2 1

PUBLISHER'S NOTE: Neither the publisher nor the author is engaged in rendering professional advice or services to the individual reader. The ideas, procedures, and suggestions contained in this book are not intended as a substitute for consulting with your physician. All matters regarding your health require medical supervision. Neither the author nor the publisher shall be liable or responsible for any loss or damage allegedly arising from any information or suggestion in this book.

Most Perigee books are available at special quantity discounts for bulk purchases for sales promotions, premiums, fund-raising, or educational use. Special books, or book excerpts, can also be created to fit specific needs. For details, write: Special Markets, Penguin Group (USA) Inc., 375 Hudson Street, New York, New York 10014.

Acknowledgments

First off, I'd like to thank my coauthor, Ben, whose calm professionalism kept me from veering off into self-indulgent ranting without stifling my idiosyncratic voice. If this book succeeds in hitting the golden mean between crazy and conformist, it's his doing.

I'd also like to thank the four women who made *The No S Diet* possible. In roughly chronological order:

My mother, whose wonderful cooking instilled a love of food in me that made the gastronomical deprivations of other diets seem intolerable. With a palate like she gave me, I had no choice but to invent my own.

My wife, Karen, who not only came up with the critical S day exception, but also served as a brutally effective front line editor. With all due respect to my actual editor and coauthor, what they saw was refined gold compared with the pre-Karen version.

Sarah Wernick, the talented, successful, and absurdly generous author of (among many others) *Strong Women*

Stay Slim, who emailed me out of the blue to encourage me to consider turning the No S Diet into a book, and then provided an unbelievable amount of practical guidance along the way. Without her, I would never have had the idea to seriously embark on this project, or known where to begin.

Our editor *ex machina*, Marian Lizzi, who picked the No S Diet out of the World Wide Wastes of the Internet and gave us a shot at the big time. I'm grateful not only for this opportunity, and for her extraordinary professional expertise, but also for her simple human kindness. To a green newbie like me, the world of publishing seemed vaguely terrifying. Marian's attentiveness and courtesy both put me at ease and inspired me to far greater focus and efficiency than any slave driver could have. You don't want to let down someone *that* nice.

But more than any particular person, I'd like to thank the members of the Nosdiet.com bulletin board—if you hadn't taken the risk of trying this crazy thing out and been generous enough to share your success stories, no one would be interested in reading a book about it.

Thank you all!
—*Reinhard*

Thanks to my parents, who taught me the importance of eating right and, whenever possible, eating well; to Doug Collar, who set me on this professional path early in life; and to Reinhard Engels, for finding simple solutions to difficult problems.

—*Ben*

Contents

3. No Sweets 61

4. No Seconds 79

5. Days That Start with S 94

6. Building the No S Habit 113

Introduction

Some time ago, I ran across a link to a website that really blew me away. It explained a diet plan that seemed so remarkable in its ease and simplicity, I was amazed everyone in the world hadn't already heard of it. Even more surprising, the creator was not a famous doctor or nutritionist or celebrity fitness guru, but a librarian-turned-computer programmer who came up with the diet because he needed to lose weight himself; and, well, it just made sense to him.

With 15 years' experience writing about health, nutrition, and weight loss for various national magazines, I was well aware that the main issue most people have with excess fat is not losing it once or twice or three times but keeping it off permanently. And while pretty much all the well-known diet plans offer effective methods for shedding pounds, they're simply too complicated, too difficult, or too unpleasant for most people to stick to over the long haul. The weight comes off...but then, sooner or later, it comes back on, too—sometimes more of it than ever.

The No S Diet is different. The list of rules is so short and simple that you can't possibly forget them. In fact, once you set the plan in motion, you barely have to think about it at all. There's no counting calories or measuring food beyond just putting it on a plate and eating it. You can have any kind of food you want (except one, and there are good reasons for that). And there's even a mechanism for breaking those few rules, and treating yourself, on a regular basis. You don't feel a desire to go off this diet, because there's nothing unpleasant about being on it.

Of course, the natural question to ask about a plan like this is, If it's so easy, how can it possibly work? We're so accustomed to diets full of deprivation, ones that leave you hungry all day or that cut out your favorite food groups, that we've come to believe weight loss and discomfort go hand in hand. But the fact is, you do eat smaller portions and consume fewer carbs, fat grams, and calories on this plan. The difference is that you barely notice it. And to judge from all the successful dieters who've happily written about their experiences on Nosdiet.com, hundreds, possibly even thousands of people have already proved that the plan works.

While I'm not usually one for writing fan letters, I contacted Reinhard and suggested we write this book together. And here we are. Regular visitors to his website will recognize the ideas in this book, which have been expanded and clarified to answer any questions you may have about a plan that is, nevertheless, just as simple and easy to follow as ever. And if you haven't heard of the No S Diet before, you're in for a nice surprise.

I'm proud to join Reinhard in presenting the No S Diet to the world. I think it's going to do a lot of people a lot of good.

—*Ben Kallen*

1

It's That Simple

THE SECRET FORMULA * EXCESS IS THE ISSUE * THREE S'S FOR THREE EXCESSES * ONE EXCEPTION * MODERATION IS THE SOLUTION * THE PROGRESS TRAP * NORMALCY CODIFIED * WHAT ABOUT NUTRITION? * WHY YOU SHOULD LISTEN TO ME * TESTIMONIALS * WHAT THE REST OF THIS BOOK IS FOR

The Secret Formula

Make everything as simple as possible, but not simpler.
—Albert Einstein

Is there really room for anything new under the sun as far as diets are concerned? Hasn't every possible gimmick already been tried—several times—without making the slightest dent in the relentless advance of obesity rates?

There's one thing left: simplicity.

The No S Diet is a diet plan so short and simple that it fits on the cover of this book. No pseudoscience, no miracle foods, no counting calories or carbs or fat or points, no disgusting recipes or draconian meal plans, just plain old common sense, charmingly and mnemonically codified. In brevity: a mantra, a haiku, a spell. But down to earth as a Kansas wheat field.

There are three rules and one exception:

* No snacks
* No sweets
* No seconds
* Except on days that start with S

And that's really all there is to it. I'm not joking. You could put this book down, walk away, and start losing weight now just by remembering those dozen-odd words. You've got the "secret formula" already.

So why keep reading?

Well, for one thing, you probably aren't quite convinced yet. Maybe you're amused, maybe you're intrigued, but you don't really believe that a huge, potentially crippling problem like being overweight or obese could be solved by a cutesy jingle. It can—by *this* cutesy jingle at least. And if you keep reading, I hope I'll convince you of that.

Excess Is the Issue

People have gotten horribly fat over the last 20 to 30 years here in America and around the world. You've heard all the shocking statistics before (see the box on the next page, if you want a refresher—they get worse every year). Why has this happened? You can follow the chain of causality endlessly; it gets infinitely complex if you pursue it far enough. But if your primary interest is in fixing the problem for yourself, the issue is actually quite simple.

✳ From 1976 to 2004, the prevalence of obesity in the United States more than doubled, from 15 percent to 32 percent of the adult population. The majority of Americans (66 percent) are now at least overweight.[1] And despite the exponential growth of the diet and "wellness" industry, the problem is only getting worse. According to Dr. John Foreyt, director of the Nutrition Research Clinic at Houston's Baylor College, "If these rates continue . . . we'll all be overweight by the year 2035 and obese by 2100."[2]

Every diet book these days starts with some sort of conspiracy theory about why people have gotten so fat. These theories generally involve evil corporations pumping us full of calories without our knowledge; the nefarious effects of mysterious stab-in-the-back substances such as refined carbohydrates, high-fructose corn syrup, and trans-fats; and the foolish and self-serving advice of the last generation of diet gurus. The reader is worked up into a state of righteous indignation: "It's not my fault that I'm fat, someone or something did this to me!" It's flattering, it's comforting, but as far as your efforts to get thin are concerned, it's dangerously wrong.

The truth is embarrassingly simpler and, well, just plain embarrassing. We're fat because we eat too much and move too little. We don't need any sneaky killer ingredients to account for our prodigious girth. Given the sheer, simple, overwhelming level of caloric intake that we as a society have become accustomed to and the paltry amount of exercise we get, it would be a miracle if we *weren't* fat. According to a 2005 report issued by the U.S. Department of Agriculture's Economic Research Service (ERS), Americans eat 16 percent more calories than they did in 1970.[3] And it's not as if they're making up for those extra calories by exercising more. In fact, according to Steven N. Blair, director of research at the Cooper Institute in Dallas, Americans burn 300 to 700 fewer calories per day than in generations past, a number that matches or even exceeds our increased food consumption.[4] Those extra calories have to go somewhere. They can't violate the first law of thermodynamics (which states that energy can never simply disappear). They are more than sufficient to account for us being as fat as we are. There is no mystery going on here.

The problem is excess, pure and simple. Corn syrup versus cane sugar, carbs versus fat, white rice versus brown rice: These are details, exciting but ultimately insignificant distractions from the giant heart of the issue: the behavior of excessive eating—or what we used to call, before we were so given to it, gluttony. Sure, some of these ingredients are suboptimal, but even if we replaced them with their more healthful equivalents we would still be consuming way too many calories and burning too few to maintain anything close to a normal weight. The issue is not ingredients. It's not a matter of replacing X with Y. It's a matter of reducing both X and Y.

Three S's for Three Excesses

No snacks, no sweets, no seconds. These restrictions aren't arbitrary—I didn't pick them just because they

✳ "The ERS food consumption (per capita) data series, one of the few series tracking long-term consumption, suggests that Americans are eating more food every year. The total amount of food available for each person to eat increased 16 percent from 1,675 pounds in 1970 to 1,950 pounds in 2003. *This increase was not isolated to a few food groups.* Fruits and vegetables also showed an increase."[5]

happen to start with the letter S (though it's certainly convenient that they do). They target the three biggest, most egregious forms of dietary excess. By cutting out these indulgences during the week, you cut out plenty, but nothing you can't comfortably do without. It's sufficient, but still humane.

The S's are easy to identify and difficult to sneak around. By eliminating snacks and seconds, you restore the obviousness of excess: Confined to a single plate at mealtime, a lot of food will *look* like a lot of food. And you don't need to do a biochemical analysis of a candy bar to know it's a sweet; you can *taste* it. With your senses on your side, self-deception becomes very difficult, and without self-deception, few of us would gorge ourselves the way we do. By following these rules, you get a good-enough idea of how much you are eating without having to pay an exorbitant and unsustainable amount of attention.

No Snacks

No snacks means no eating between meals. Until very recently, this would have been a no-brainer, but now everyone seems to be convinced that snacking is good for you. And it does seem to be the case that under laboratory conditions, people who eat a controlled amount of calories over the course of many small meals metabolize them *slightly* more efficiently than people who eat the same amount of calories in the traditional three.[6] But in real-world conditions, people who snack wind up eating a lot more food; so despite a slightly faster metabolism, they chunk up. The No S Diet isn't a lab diet, biology divorced from psychology. It's a real-world diet, built to withstand the pressures of your stubborn, sneaky mind.

Do snackers really eat more? Astonishingly more. According to data from the Continuing Surveys of Food Intake by Individuals, conducted by the U.S. Department of Agriculture (USDA), over 90 percent of our increased calorie consumption since 1977 has come from increased between-meal eating.[7] If this statistic is accurate, snacking is not only the biggest problem in terms of dietary excess but is almost the *entire* problem.

If you think about it, it makes sense that snackers eat more. The trouble with eating frequently throughout the day is that it's impossible to get a sense of how much you are consuming without paying an exorbitant amount of attention, such as counting calories or points. Doing all that math is way too much conscious overhead to sustain for the long term, and it's not something you can automate into unconscious habit. You stop paying attention because it's too much work, and when you stop paying attention you eat too much, without even realizing it.

The less often you eat, the fewer calories you consume.

—David Levitsky, Ph.D., professor of nutritional
sciences at Cornell University[8]

No Sweets

No sweets is the only rule that targets a specific substance (all most diets do), but there is a critical difference from the usual dietary substance prohibitions.
Because you are allowed to eat sweets on weekends
and holidays (the S days), this rule is not so much a
prohibition as a recasting of sweets from the routine
staple they have become to their traditional role as
"desserts," something deserved, a treat, an incentive,
a reward. It's really more about behavior than substance, about turning the weakness of a sweet tooth
into a motivating strength. Viewed this way, the No
S Diet is really profoundly pro-sweet: Deserved desserts really do taste much better. On S days, you can
enjoy sweets without guilt, without also hating them
for what they are doing to your body. You can plan
and anticipate something much better than what you'd
get by opportunistically raiding the fridge. Temptation
becomes incentive.

Note that the rule is *no sweets*, not no sugar. Sweets
are defined as something whose principal source of
calories is added sugar (whether refined or natural):
cookies, Pop-Tarts, cola, candy bars, and so on. You
don't have to go checking lists of ingredients and driving waiters crazy; your taste buds will let you know.

If you have to wonder (for example, yogurt or peanut butter), it's probably okay. By targeting just the really egregious offenders, you'll be cutting out a significant amount of calories. And when you avoid making yourself crazy over borderline foods, you'll be that much more likely to stick with the plan. The clear-cut cases are 80 percent of the problem and 0 percent of the headache.

Do we eat enough sugar that avoiding sweets during the week will make a decisive difference? Sadly, yes, more than enough. We eat more than 10 times as much added sugar as our nineteenth-century ancestors did.[9] That's a lot of sugar calories and a lot of room for improvement. So much room that we could still enjoy plenty of sugar—say, merely five times as much as our ancestors—and still lose weight. Given the magnitude of excess in our current level of sugar consumption, there is no reason to resort to sweeping deprivations, denying ourselves carbs in general or even all sugar. No sweets during the week is enough—and it's sustainable.

No Seconds
No seconds means that at each meal you limit yourself to eating the food that is on one physical plate. Fill it up once, and then no refills. Yes, you can fit a lot onto a plate, but you can't do it without seeing that it's a lot. That gentle pressure on your eyeballs is surprisingly effective. In the beginning, some whopping plates are to be expected. That's okay. The important thing is to build the habit and eat enough to see you through to your next meal without snacking. In time, you'll get

very good at budgeting just how much it takes to do this without hunger or excess. If it costs you a few extra calories in the form of big firsts up front to buy the habit of structured mealtime eating, they're calories well spent.

Do people who stick with single-plate meals really eat less than people who go back for seconds or thirds? According to an experiment conducted by Brian Wansink at the Cornell University Food and Brand Lab, single-platers ate an average of 14 percent less per meal, despite the fact that they took much bigger initial portions.[10]

One Exception

Each of these rules on its own would probably help you lose weight. And taken together, they ensure that you won't compensate for eating less in one area by eating more in another. But losing weight is only part of the issue. Keeping the weight off is just as important, and usually far more difficult. Moderate as the rules just described are, you probably couldn't adhere to them 7 days a week, 365 days a year, without feeling

✳ I'll be talking a lot about "days that start with S" in this book, and since that's a bit of a mouthful, I'll usually refer to them as S days. I'll refer to "days that do NOT start with S" (even more of a mouthful) as N days (i.e., NON-S days). You can also think of "N days" as standing for "*normal* days."

deprived and resentful. That's where the critical No S Diet exception comes in.

It works like this: On days that start with the letter S you are free to eat whatever you like: snacks, sweets, seconds—you name it. The training wheels come off.

There are two kinds of S days: days of the week that actually start with the letter S (Saturday and Sunday) and special days. Special days include (your) national and (your) religious holidays, and the birthdays of (your) close family and friends. You probably wouldn't have dieted on the special days anyway, but with the No S Diet, you don't have to feel guilty about it.

S days are a necessary safety valve, an incentive, and a reward. They aren't binge days; binging comes from resentment, and who resents reward? And your weekday habits will start to carry over to the weekends. Less will seem like more; and gradually, without any conscious intervention, you'll eat less.

These three rules and one exception may be simple, but they're sharp. They target the right problem—excess—with the right solution—moderation.

Moderation Is the Solution

Given that the problem is excess, you would think it would be obvious that the solution is moderation. But

---

✳ No S Diet targets the right problem—excess—with the right solution—moderation.

somehow all other diet plans seem to have missed this connection. They try to cope with the issue of excessive eating by proposing another, equal and opposite excess: either an excess of attention (counting stuff) or an excess of deprivation (restricting whole categories of foods). They try to solve one problem by introducing another.

I call the excess of attention diets *substance-accounting diets* and the excess of deprivation diets *forbidden-foods diets*. I'll consider each in turn, because I think the virtues of the No S Diet become obvious in comparison.

Substance-accounting diets are plans in which you count calories, carbs, fat, points, whatever—some quantifiable substance. The appeal of these diets is you can eat whatever you want, as long as you "balance the books" at some point. You can eat a lot now, as long as you make up for it later. It's like an accountant's ledger.

These diets tend to fail because balancing the books is too much work. It requires you to pay an exorbitant and unsustainable amount of attention. It's not something you can automate into unconscious habit. Eventually, some stress or distraction is going to come along, and you're just not going to be able to spare the mental energy that tracking every bite requires.

It's also not fun. I use the word *accounting* instead of counting not just because it's job-like in the amount of time it takes but because I want to emphasize that this is profoundly boring. Much like being a financial accountant. No offense to any accountants out there, but I assume that you wouldn't be in that line of work unless you were getting (well) paid.

The forbidden-foods diets have this Manichean, dualist, view of the world. There are good foods and evil foods. Carbs and fat are the two biggies, alternating roles depending on the system. You can eat as much as you want of the good foods as long as you don't go anywhere near the evil foods. The appeal is you can go on being a glutton as long as you confine your gluttony to the good foods. All you have to do is focus your excessive eating. The downside is you really, really start to miss the evil foods. And because you're basically still a glutton—you haven't learned to moderate your appetites, just to redirect them—you're not especially good at resisting what you want and eventually you break down.

According to some diet authorities, the reason forbidden-foods diets initially seem to work is simply because people get sick and tired of eating the same old thing all the time and so they start eating less. And these diets really do work, for a while. People starting on these diets often do eat less and lose weight. But not for the reason they think. And not for long. Because it's not that the good foods are really any better; it's just that the simple boredom and disgust of being on such a monotonous diet makes people eat less. And, of course, boredom and disgust are also the reason most people eventually give up. So the reason these diets initially work is also the reason they ultimately fail: Their strength *is* their weakness. In recognition of this underlying, flawed mechanism, it might be more accurate to call these plans "disgusting-food diets."

The advantages of the No S Diet over forbidden-foods and substance-accounting diets are pretty obvious, I think. There are no sweeping, categorical restrictions as with the forbidden-foods diets; you can eat anything you want, at the appropriate time. It's basically, on one level, a shortcut to caloric restriction, a way of getting a sense of how much you are eating without the tedium of having to keep an exact count. You can get a good-enough approximation of the amount you're eating without getting bogged down in all that substance-accounting detail. With substance-accounting diets, just *finding* the excess is most of the work. On the No S Diet, finding excess is no work at all—it jumps right out at you. When you limit your caloric input opportunities to three single-plate meals a day, it's *obvious* when you are eating too much. You don't have to count, you can *see* it. And because you haven't wasted most of your energy just looking for excess, you're in much better condition to confront it.

The Progress Trap

Pretty much any diet will lose you weight if you stick with it; the problem is, you won't. According to the U.S. Food and Drug Administration (FDA), 95 percent of dieters fail to stick with their diets for more than a few months.[11] And is it any wonder? Popular diets are heavily optimized for rapid progress. They may be effective in an abstract, biochemical sense, but they don't take human psychology and motivation into account and are, therefore, extremely difficult and unpleasant to be on for any length of time. Even if you could lose "9 pounds of belly fat in 11 days," as a ubiquitous Internet ad promises, what would you do afterward? If maintenance gets any attention at all from these plans it's as an afterthought, a "Phase 2" tucked away in the back of the book that hardly anyone ever gets to. But maintenance is more important than progress. Progress is intrinsically temporary; maintenance is what you'll be doing the rest of your life.

The No S Diet gives maintenance its proper focus. It does this by treating weight control as a mental problem, not a physical one. It focuses on incentives and enforceability, on leveraging limited reserves of willpower to build sustainable habits. The simple, natural, unobtrusive behaviors it prescribes soon become automatic. Unlike most diets, which get more and more insufferable as the gimmick ages, the No S Diet gets progressively easier. Instead of fighting against bad eating habits or pretending they don't exist, you develop good eating habits, which soon start to carry you along.

Ask yourself if you can imagine staying on a particular diet for the rest of your life. If not, don't bother starting; it's a waste of time and will.

Even (especially!) successful dieters from other systems will find the No S Diet attractive. "What next?" isn't a hypothetical question for them, and chances are "more of the same" is not an appealing answer. Successful dieters are in a better position to see the deficiencies of their diets *because* they succeeded. A unsuccessful dieter might think, "If only I'd tried harder!" It's

---

✳ You will lose weight on pretty much any diet if you stick with it; the problem is, you won't.

difficult for someone who hasn't made progress to appreciate how much harder and more important maintenance is; it's impossible not to appreciate for someone who has.

A big reason the No S Diet is so sustainable is that it is actually *enjoyable*. It isn't just less awful than other diets, a slightly more bearable grind toward a distant goal. It will actually make you enjoy food more. On the No S Diet, no pleasure is denied, just delayed and contained. Served up on the platter of limited opportunity, each pleasure becomes even more pleasurable than it was before. Maybe you wouldn't do it *solely* for pleasure, but you can do it *also* for pleasure. And when the goal is distant and doubtful, or boring because already (temporarily) attained, that makes all the difference.

Forbidden-food diets like low-carb or low-fat fail miserably in this regard. At the outset, it might seem worth it to trade pasta for unlimited steaks (or vice versa), but it gets old fast. Diet programs like Weight Watchers that require you to be a full-time calorie (or carb, or fat, or point) accountant are time-consuming and joyless. Besides the sheer tedium of compliance, if you come to think of food as fuel, a mere quantity, you'll come to loathe it *and* your number crunching-munching self.

Long-term weight management has not only been an *unsolved* problem but a largely *unconsidered* one. Being overweight tends to be seen as some kind of temporary emergency requiring drastic intervention—a manifestly ridiculous view, but apparently good enough to sustain a multibillion-dollar industry. A few marketing departments have taken to peppering their quick-fix promises with talk of "lifestyles" and "ways of eating," but that's rare and superficial—doublespeak to counter obvious objections rather than real solutions. Almost no one has seriously considered how to recast a temporary emergency into its opposite: sustainable normalcy.

Normalcy Codified

The No S Diet is simple and specific. Commercial diets are too complicated for people with outside interests to follow (eating = math). Conventional-wisdom rules about diet are too simplistic and vague to be useful (eat only when you're hungry). The No S Diet finds the happy medium between the two, the right level of abstraction. You have just enough direction to do your job but not so much that you resent its imposition. You have a solid framework, but the details are up to you. You have sufficient guidance and sufficient freedom. It's a system without too much system.

I'm not going to lie to you: The No S Diet *is* a diet, a bunch of rules about how you should eat. But the idea is that the rules are simple and intuitive and natural enough that they'll eventually become habit, second nature. They'll start out rational and become routine. A member of the Nosdiet.com bulletin board put it beautifully:

> *A month in, I don't think I'm on a diet anymore. I'm just eating normally, but it's a different normally than a month ago. There's nothing left to stick*

to; eating because I'm bored is unsatisfying now, going for seconds leaves me feeling uncomfortably full, and sweets that aren't treats are nowhere near as satisfying as they used to be.

When you are trying to form a new habit—to make something second nature—it helps if it jibes with your "first nature." It will be easier to learn and have fewer unintended side effects. When I explain the No S Diet to naturally thin people, they often have trouble understanding what the big deal is. "But that's what I do already, more or less," they tell me. I'm not offended; on the contrary, I take this as the highest compliment, as evidence that the No S Diet is just the explicit formulation of something natural and widespread, or, at least, formerly natural and widespread.

The No S Diet is a lot like the way naturally thin people, across societies and times and cultures, have always eaten. The details vary a little from place to place, and it's never been formulated *exactly* like the No S Diet, but a limited number of limited-size meals, with sweets and big feasts reserved for special occasions, is a pretty universal way of eating. And remember, being thin is not some anomalous condition found only among Okinawans and French women and Paleolithic cavemen. Most people in most places at most times in history were thin, even here in the United States, until very recently—around 1980. So you don't need to look for some crazy, far-out solution. Just eat like they did. It's safe, it's a known quantity, we know how to do it, it clearly works; and doing something this normal is going to be easier than doing something strange and historically unprecedented. The behavior of thousands of generations of your ancestors has carved deep grooves for these habits to fall into.

The year 1980 is obviously an arbitrary cutoff, but you get the point. It's close; it's not strange. Many of you reading this book can (or should be able to) remember 1980. Nor do you have to replicate the 1980 diet in every extraneous detail. No S is all the time machine you need.

People talk about the "French paradox," the idea that the French can eat fatty, carby, delicious food and still stay skinny, while health-conscious, calorie-counting Americans are the fattest people on earth. It seems not only improbable but unjust. The French love their food and stay skinny; we hate our food and get fat.

Sometimes red wine or olive oil or some other miracle ingredient is held to account for this. But the thing is, this phenomenon is not so particularly French. As I mentioned before, look to any country in which meals and meal times are still largely governed by tradition, and you'll find the same thing: People make their food choices based on custom and taste instead of health and somehow stay thin. Japan is often held up as another example of this. And the Japanese also have miracle foods. But their miracle foods are completely different from the French miracle foods. And keep in mind that obesity rates in most places where American-style eating hasn't become entrenched are closer to those of France and Japan than to ours.

What do all these countries have in common? Not miracle foods. We're the schmucks who believe in miracle foods. What they have in common are traditional structures around how and when people eat. The details may differ a little from country to country, but there is a surprising degree of overlap. Traditional eaters don't permasnack; they eat discrete, social meals. Treats and excesses exist, but they're reserved for special feast days.

Fortunately, we haven't lost all of our traditional eating behaviors. Eating is still an inherently social activity. Even in modern times, we have customs that involve eating meals in groups, with family or friends. We tend not to eat meals alone.

So why is it that no other diet plan seems to consider this obvious and important fact? It's bad enough that you yourself have to eat the nasty fare these diets prescribe; there's no way you're going to succeed if you have to convince others to eat it too or if you have to cook separate meals. The No S Diet dispenses with all that. You eat normal food, just like the people you're eating with. You just eat less of it. They don't even have to know you're doing anything different. No more separate meals. No more awkward excuses at dinner parties. No more family members secretly or not-so-secretly hoping you'll get it over with and fail already so they can go back to eating normal food again. Who needs this extra stress? Dieting is hard enough without having to convince other people to go along with it.

In the end, the No S Diet is really just the explicit formulation of the implicit, traditional rules that used to govern our eating and still do in some places: normalcy codified. It's not exactly the same, but it's close enough to resonate deeply and simple enough to be easily replicable.

✳ In borrowing from a food culture, pay attention to how a culture eats, as well as to what it eats. In the case of the French paradox, it may not be the dietary nutrients that keep the French healthy (lots of saturated fat and alcohol?!) so much as the dietary habits: small portions, no seconds or snacking, communal meals—and the serious pleasure taken in eating. (Worrying about diet can't possibly be good for you.) Let culture be your guide, not science.

—Michael Pollan, author of *The Omnivore's Dilemma*[12]

What About Nutrition?

The No S Diet is a framework for controlling excess. Beyond that it makes no stipulations about your nutritional or gastronomic choices. That doesn't mean they're not important; they're just separate issues. Fight one enemy at a time, not three at once.

That said, I find that having a limited number of limited-quantity meals makes me take each one more seriously, from both a gastronomic and a nutritional point of view. Pretty much every meal I eat is delicious or healthy or both. Each plate is a spotlight. You can't help but think about taste and nutrition because you know you have only three meals a day and only one chance to do each meal right. You've raised the stakes, made each input opportunity important—something to be taken advantage of. You'll eat healthier, more delicious meals without further explicit, systematic intervention.

It should also be mentioned that simple excess, and not the lack of any particular dietary substance, is the most pressing nutritional problem today. The single healthiest thing most of us could do today from a nutritional standpoint, *by a long shot*, would be simply to eat less. You have no business worrying about antioxidants when you're 50 pounds overweight.

Why You Should Listen to Me

I am neither a doctor, a nurse, a dietitian, a nutritionist, a personal trainer, nor any other kind of health professional. *I am not an expert.* This is a tremendous advantage.

Diet is not a problem that requires specialized knowledge. It is a general problem with an obvious solution. If I were encumbered by any form of expertise, this obviousness wouldn't be nearly as striking. A doctor cannot convincingly say, *"Duh."*

I am a librarian by training and a computer programmer by accident. A few years ago, I noticed I was getting a little too heavy (borderline obese, actually, if you want to get technical) and came up with this cute, commonsense formula. To give credit where credit is due, I think it was my wife who came up with the critical "days that start with S" exception (she claims not to remember this). I had no expectation that it would actually work, but within two months I'd lost 20 pounds. There was no pain and suffering, there were no unbearable pangs of hunger; I barely even noticed what I was doing—all I noticed was that I wasn't feeling disgusted and guilty from stuffing myself all the time anymore.

I've since lost an additional 20 pounds (so my total progress has been from 210 to 170, or 40 pounds down from where I started and 50 pounds down from my all-time high of 220). To be fair, that second drop may have something to do with the fact that I also started doing some exercise (see page 173). This seems to be my natural, healthy weight, 10 or 15 pounds below what I imagined my ideal weight should be when I started. People now describe me as lean, which is sweet music to a lifelong "husky."

I've been on the diet since March 2002, with no yo-yoing. Unlike most diets that get more and more insufferable as the gimmick ages, the No S Diet gets progressively easier and becomes largely unconscious. It becomes almost like a religious dietary restriction: effortlessly inviolable. (You don't see a whole subgenre of books geared at strictly observant Jews and Muslims on the theme of how to avoid stuffing your face with pork and shellfish.)

People I explained it to responded enthusiastically, and so I decided to stick it on the web. I'm a computer programmer, so that seemed like a natural thing to do. And I've been astonished at the response. I thought the No S Diet would be interesting just as a personal record of what one guy did. But people took this idiosyncratic, personal, and admittedly kind of crazy-sounding system and applied it to their own problems—successfully. Even more successfully than I had, in some cases, because they had more weight to lose.

* The No S Diet gets progressively easier and becomes largely unconscious.

Testimonials

Hundreds of people took the risk of making a major life decision based on the advice of a guy with no relevant credentials, with no authority beyond that which comes from making sense; and it paid off. (And these are just the hundreds that I know about; not everyone who does the No S Diet sends me email me or posts to the website's bulletin board—much as I wish they would.) You readers of this book are luckier than those bold early adopters. You don't have to rely on the No S Diet merely making sense; you also have the experience of this first generation of beta testers to guide you. In this section I present a small sample of what people have to say about the diet; see the Nosdiet.com bulletin board for many more.

Because readers are presumably most interested in blood-and-guts numbers, pounds lost are given in **bold** for each testimonial. It's not the only metric, it's not the best metric (see page 134), but it's the metric everybody seems to want to see. And if nothing else, it is evidence that significant weight can be lost on the No S Diet, which, given the obvious moderation and sustainability of this approach, is perhaps the more incredible part.

At **96 pounds** down, Josie from Washington is probably our reigning pound-for-pound champ. She writes:

I have been dieting and following this program seriously for nine months. In that time, I have lost an incredible amount of weight and increased fitness in ways I never dreamed possible. I started off at 289 pounds. I am now at 193 and still dropping.... This plan really, truly works! Be kind to yourself. Some days are just better than others. Do the best you can and Stick With It!...I cheat every weekend!! I love red wines and dark beer! This diet allows me that choice. I truly believe my finding this diet has changed my life forever. No words can express my thanks! My doctor is going to go into shock when I go see him in October! What fun!! Yippee!

Brian from Ireland writes:

I started this sometime last summer or fall, can't remember exactly. I lost **40–50 pounds** *and seem to be holding steady around 185 pounds for several months now, which is good for my height and I'm happy with it. I'm still doing No S; it seems once I got to my ideal weight I stopped losing more.*

Sensible, balanced eating. No way-out menus. I love it! I've never felt so content about my weight or my appetite.

Deb from Long Island writes:

I eat what I enjoy, and I balance that with regular exercise....I would rather take longer to get slim than feel like I'm in a biochemical war with my food....I love it all....It's almost my first-year anniversary with No S and I have lost about **17 pounds....**

I will never ever switch from this life plan....It is foolproof.

Rich from Toronto, who has since lost over **30 pounds**, writes:

A month in, I don't think I'm on a diet anymore. I'm just eating normally, but it's a different normally than a month ago. There's nothing left to stick to. Eating because I'm bored is unsatisfying now, going for seconds leaves me feeling uncomfortably full, and sweets that aren't treats are nowhere near as satisfying as they used to be.

James from Maine writes:

*I've been doing No S since last June. I don't know my exact starting weight, but my best guess is that I'm down about **40 or 50 pounds** since then. I still have a long way to go (probably at least 75 more pounds), but after eight months I'm smaller than I've been in well over a decade, my belt has a half-dozen new notches cut into it, I have more energy, and I don't get as tired.*

Perhaps more important, my relationship with food has been repaired. I now know what it is to enjoy food, both while I'm actually eating it, and when the act of eating it lingers in my memory. No more binge-guilt cycles. No more "I shouldn't be eating this...." I just follow the rules, and enjoy the abundance of tasty, nutritious food in my life.

Spiralstares from New York writes:

I started the No S Diet in the middle of June; now almost exactly five months later I am down

50 pounds. *So it's been my experience that No S really works if you commit to it.*

Emma from an undisclosed location writes:

*I looked through my diary this morning and counted 10 weeks No S. (Smile) How time flies! I've lost 4.5 kg [*10 pounds*].*

Prior to No S I was a constant grazer with an insatiable sweet tooth, and despite regular exercise I was gradually getting fatter. I felt depressed and guilty about the way I was eating. I reached the upper threshold of my healthy weight range, and I'd be officially overweight now if I hadn't found No S and this board.

Kathleen from Brisbane, Australia, writes:

*I started in mid-2005. Over 18 months, I've lost 27 kg [*59.4 pounds*]—from 111 down to 84. [244.2 down to 184]. Cool. My BMI, for what that's worth, has dropped from 35 to 26.5. I haven't been doing much exercise beyond walking to the train station.*

SilentButDeftly from Boston writes:

Does it work? Yes!

12 pounds *since November and still losing. Only about a pound a week, but they're not coming back. It can be the easiest thing in the world to do, but there are times when it's almost frustratingly difficult. I can tell you it's worth it—I've never before had anyone ask me if I'd lost weight without wanting a favor. People are starting to notice, and they're amazed when I tell them that I'm still eating what I used to eat, just less of it.*

Rhumba from San Francisco writes:

*Yippee!! I just reached the **20-pound** weight-loss mark. I checked on the member list to see how long it has been. I joined in June, so the loss is about 1 pound per week, or a teensy bit more.*

I think of all the diets, exercise programs, personal trainers, and general misery I went through over so many years with little result, and this simple, easy system works so well.

Navin from Kentucky writes:

*I'm another example of the "slow loser." I've been doing this over two years, and I've lost about 1 pound a month.... While it doesn't sound like much, do the math and it adds up over time, as I'm down about **26 pounds**.*

The fast loss of other diets is fool's gold. Sticking with it is the bane of any diet, I'm sure all of us know more people who have lost big, and then gained it right back, than who have lost weight and kept it off for any length of time....

Unless you are morbidly obese, a slow, steady, maintainable loss is a good thing. Your body will thank you later.

Catbert from "Planet Texas" writes:

*I've been No-S-ing for about 11 months now and just recently hit the **25-pound** mark—too cool! My husband reminded me the other day I should let you all in on my success. I'm still No-S-ing, still walking and still losing. It doesn't get much better than this!*

Kevin from Maryland writes:

*Since June, [I lost] about **20 pounds**, but most of that in the first three months.*

At this point, I'm closing in on my ideal weight (probably another 10 or so). Before I started resistance exercise, I had actually weighed about five pounds less. I might not make it all the way down to my ideal weight given that I eat whatever non-sweet, one-plate meal I want, three times a day.

When you stop and think about it, by world standards, that's still a pretty generous amount of food.

At 46, I'm 10 pounds over what I graduated college at, and I'm significantly stronger, although I know I couldn't run as far or as fast as I could then.

Do it. You'll love it.

Not that mere popularity should sway you, but the website, which I proudly run out of my basement on a hobbyist's budget, is now linked to by thousands of other websites and blogs and is consistently among the most popular entries on social bookmarking sites like del.icio.us and directories such as Yahoo!, outplacing presumably much-better-funded commercial plans.

As a phenomenon, it's become a little like the diet equivalent of that cold-prevention drug Airborne, which proudly boasts that it was "made by a teacher." For people tired of being let down by experts, the fact that the No S Diet was created by a librarian seems to have had a similar appeal.

What the Rest of This Book Is For

Convinced yet? I hope so. But perhaps you're still a little confused. That's what the rest of this book is for.

Maybe you have questions about how precisely to interpret some of the rules. Is a snack defined as when you eat, or is it a particular kind of food (see page 36)? Does fruit count as a sweet (see page 75)? Is there any limit as to how many sweets, snacks, and seconds I can eat on days that start with S (see page 99)?

I've been astonished by the number of questions my simple, clear formula has elicited since I posted it to the web in March 2002. In Chapters 2 through 5, you'll find answers to the most frequently asked questions, including the ones I just listed, organized logically by the rule (or exception) to which they pertain. Skim over the rules chapters in the middle of the book to clear up any compliance questions you may have (some of which may not have occurred to you yet—so do take a look, even if you can't think of any at the moment).

Then I'd suggest carefully reading Chapter 6, "Building the No S Habit." The No S rules are powerful, and very habit-friendly, the carrot and stick you need to train your eating behaviors. But just as a trainer of wild animals wouldn't step into the ring without first knowing something about the animals in his or her charge, you should familiarize yourself with the nature of the habits you are about to train. Besides big-picture philosophical stuff, Chapter 6 also contains useful, practical advice on setting milestones and recovering from failures—the nitty-gritty on whipping your habits into shape.

This is a spare, minimalist diet, and I've tried to keep the book that way too. In Chapter 7, "Beyond the No S Diet," you'll read about all the peripheral issues and fluff I've tried to keep out of the rest of this book. You might be surprised at some of the issues I consider peripheral (like nutrition) and fluff (recipes). *Beyond* doesn't (necessarily) mean "bad"; and Chapter 7 also contains a discussion of how you might apply the principles behind the No S Diet to other self-improvement projects (like exercise) as well as a brief description of the free online resources at Nosdiet.com.

2

No Snacks

WHY MEALS ARE GOOD AND SNACKS ARE BAD * WHY SNACKERS EAT MORE * SNACKERS EAT MORE OF THE WORST KINDS OF STUFF * ARE SNACKS *WHEN* I EAT OR *WHAT* I EAT? * WHAT MAKES A MEAL A MEAL? * SNACKING IS NOT NORMAL * MAKING EXCESS VISIBLE * WHY IS EVERYONE ELSE SO PRO-SNACK? * WHY DO PEOPLE SNACK SO MUCH MORE THAN THEY USED TO? * AREN'T SNACKS METABO-LIZED MORE EFFICIENTLY THAN MEALS? * WHAT ABOUT HEALTHY SNACKS? * WHAT ABOUT DIET BARS? * SNACKING IS BAD FOR YOUR TEETH! * WHAT IF I GET HUNGRY BETWEEN MEALS? * ISN'T IT BETTER TO EAT WHEN I'M HUNGRY? * WHAT IF I'M NOT HUNGRY AT MEALTIME? * IS IT EXTRA-GOOD TO EAT FEWER MEALS? * DO DRINKS COUNT AS SNACKS? * DOES IT MATTER WHEN I EAT MY MEALS? * WHAT IF MY DOCTOR SAYS I NEED TO EAT MORE THAN THREE MEALS A DAY? * WHAT IF I HAVE A CRAZY SCHEDULE? * BUT THIN PEOPLE SOMETIMES SNACK

Why Meals Are Good and Snacks Are Bad

No snacks is probably the most contentious rule. Every-one nowadays seems to want us to eat between meals, from the junk-food manufacturers who produce billions of dollars of snack foods each year to the health-food gurus, who are more often than not pushing their own brands of snack products.

And it's not as if snacking even needed the sanction of all these authorities—it's plenty appealing on its own. Snacking is convenient. Most snack foods take no time to prepare: Just unwrap and start chewing. There's no time lost even in consuming them; we don't have to sit down at the table, we can multitask, snacking while we are working or driving or relaxing in front of the television. And there are no dishes to do afterward. Snack foods are cheap. Snacking protects us from the mild discomfort of ever feeling hungry. And then, of course, to top it all off, diet gurus tell us that many small snacks are metabolized more efficiently than a few big meals, so we can feel virtuous for doing what we'd do anyway.

But consider this: Back when we as a society were skinny, we didn't really eat snacks. When we stuck with three meals a day, more or less, we were thin. It was only when family meal structures broke down in the 1980s and we started snacking in earnest that obesity rates skyrocketed. According to U.S. Department of Agriculture (USDA) studies, over 90 percent of the increase in calorie consumption from 1977 to 1996 came from snacks.[1] So, snacks are not just the number one problem in terms of overconsumption, they are almost the *entire* problem.

What's more, it wasn't the *size* of individual snacks that increased, but their *frequency*—the "grazing" that diet gurus love to praise. As Harvard economist David M. Cutler pointed out in his 2003 paper interpreting these data: "The average number of snacks increased by 60 percent over this period, thus more snacks per day—rather than more calories per snack—account for the majority of the increase in the calories from snacks."[2] So, although it might be tempting for some to keep snacking frequently while focusing on making those snacks smaller or healthier as a way to reduce total snack calories, there is no historical precedent for such behavior. We didn't get fat because we ate bigger or less healthy snacks; we got fat simply because we ate *more* snacks. So it makes sense to do the opposite, to eat fewer snacks, like we used to. We know how to do that; we know we can; and we know it works.

Now, I don't like to put too much weight on any one study. But this is a pretty authoritative source, and 90 percent gives us quite a bit of wiggle room. And the bulk of studies on the subject of snacking and weight gain confirm the association. Even if it were only half true, if "only" 45 percent of our excess calories came from snacks, that would still be more than sufficient justification to act.

Why Snackers Eat More

Whatever the exact percentages, it's clear that people who snack frequently eat more than people who don't—a lot more. Why is this?

It makes obvious sense if you think about it a bit. If you are a snacker, you eat more because more input opportunities means it is impossible to monitor how much you are eating without paying an exorbitant and unsustainable amount of attention. You simply have no idea how much you are eating. Your eyes, which used to be able to see excess when it was concentrated in a few discrete meals, are now useless. You are literally eating blind. Lots of small quantities, each of which looks small and harmless in itself, are smuggled past your eyes, invisibly adding up to a huge amount. Instead of having to keep watch just three meals day, you always have to be on guard. That's too much work, so most of us soon give up and are overrun.

When you snack, the only way you can get a handle on how much you are eating is to *count* (calories, carbs, points, whatever), a totally unnatural, unpleasant, and unsustainable activity. You are enabling one unnatural activity (snacking) by introducing another (counting). And because counting is unsustainably hard, while snacking is the easiest thing in the world, you'll probably soon be left with just snacking—except now the habit will be reinforced by the idea that snacking can (theoretically) be managed.

Snackers Eat More of the Worst Kinds of Stuff

Snackers don't just eat more, they also tend to eat more of the worst kinds of stuff: highly processed, highly caloric prepackaged food products. So greater input frequency goes hand in hand with greater caloric density—a double whammy. Pro-snackers like to talk of their habit as grazing, but animals that graze eat *grass*, not candy bars. Most people who graze go about it like chocaholic lions; it would be more accurate to call it high-frequency *gorging*.

It makes sense that snack food tends to be like this. People snack in large part because snack foods are cheap and filling and convenient. A huge industry has sprung up around optimizing foods for these qualities, at the expense of any nutritional value besides mere calories. So if you snack, not only are you eating blind but you're eating blind in a room full of booby traps. You *could* eat healthy snacks, but most of us, most of the time, don't. Chances are you'll eat the processed snack foods that have been *optimized* for snacking at the expense of nutrition—why wouldn't you? They embody the real reasons you snack. Most of us wouldn't be snacking to begin with if it weren't for the existence of such temptingly cheap, convenient, highly caloric foods; and we didn't, before they existed. A token healthy carrot or celery stick now and then accomplishes nothing except the legitimization of an otherwise unhealthy and self-destructive behavior. Your healthy carrot is a pretext. Save it for a meal.

I don't want to emphasize this "qualitative" part of the argument against snacks too strongly, because the USDA study cited earlier suggests that snacking

---

✳ The USDA data has some surprising implications. Despite all the prominent moaning about the ill effects of eating out all the time and supersized portions, the amount of calories consumed during meals has stayed roughly the same since 1977. So while it is true that we eat a higher percentage of our meal calories at fast-food joints, that doesn't translate into more total calories: McDonald's has not, it seems, made us fat. Fun as it may be to cast stones at the fast-food industry, if this data is accurate, we'll have to find some other culprit.

frequency rather than size is the real problem. Snacks may be bad, but they've always been bad—they're just a lot more frequent now.

Are Snacks *When* I Eat or *What* I Eat?

For the purposes of the No S Diet, snacks are *when*, not *what*. Pretzels with lunch are lunch. Maybe not a particularly healthy lunch, but the No S Diet delegates that micro-decision to you. A snack, for No S Diet purposes, is any food you eat between meals. A meal is any food you eat at meals. The *kind* of food is completely up to you.

That being said, you will probably wind up eating a lot less unhealthy snack food. Why? Because you'll feel silly eating snacks for meals. They're in the wrong conceptual category. You'll want meal foods for meals; and that's great, because as I just pointed out, snack foods tend to be terrible for you. In this way, you indirectly limit the *what* with the *when*.

Conversely, of course, eating foods that you would normally eat at a meal (like a salad or a sandwich) between meals still counts as a snack. So there's no getting around this rule by eating a steak au poivre on your coffee break instead of a bag of chips.

What Makes a Meal a Meal?

I'm going to keep this real simple: Define the term *meal* however you like, as long as you get only three of them a day (or some similarly small predetermined number; see page 58). It's important to keep this definition as clear as possible, or you'll be tempted to wiggle around it.

That being said, inserting a little bit of formality around mealtimes can be a great help. If you make meals feel distinct and separate from the rest of your activities, you'll teach your appetite to associate eating with these external signs, and not others. In his famous experiment, Ivan Pavlov trained his dogs to salivate at the sound of a bell by ringing it before feedings. Your mealtime rituals can have the same associative power. If you practice them consistently, you'll feel strange eating without them. You'll condition yourself to get hungry only when the time and circumstances are right.

Here are some ideas to get you started: Eat at the table instead of at your desk or on the couch. Never eat while you are doing something else, like watching TV or driving or working at the computer. Eat with others when possible. Say grace. Punctuate the end of each meal by brushing your teeth. Even little things like an attractive place setting can make a difference.

The more you use little marks of attention like these to distinguish mealtimes from the rest of the day, the more "sacred" you make your mealtimes. The more your unconscious mind is impressed, the firmer the association between mealtimes and eating becomes and the less hungry you'll be between meals. You'll also come to see meals as something positive to look forward to and not as a restraint. Making meals feel special isn't a requirement of the No S Diet, but it can make things a lot easier, and it's not a bad thing in itself.

Snacking Is Not Normal

The convenience of packaged snack foods, their biggest selling point, is in fact a dangerous liability. These snacks are so tempting, not because they are so good but because they are so *easy*. They require so little time or work or money—or *attention*. The bar to enjoying a candy bar is very, very low. You can trip over it, it's so low. It's barely a decision. It's almost a default.

It used to be the opposite. Food used to be very, very inconvenient to prepare. Food was expensive and hard to preserve. You couldn't just whip out a Power-Bar when you needed an extra boost to plow the field. Almost everyone spent almost all their time preparing food: planting it, growing it, harvesting it, hunting it, cooking it. When people sat down to eat the food they'd just spent most of their waking hours preparing, it was a big deal. It was a social event. It was formal. It was distinct from the rest of the day. It was eaten with real gratitude. It was a meal.

So despite what the snack-food industry and their diet guru cohorts would have you believe, eating only during meals is profoundly normal, nothing you should be afraid of. It's snacking that is the weird, anomalous behavior that needs justifying, that only people in fat societies indulge in.

Sticking with meals has cultural breadth as well as historical depth. It is a cross-cultural practice. They do it in France. They do it in China. We used to do it right here in the United States. You don't have to look to some far-off place in the distant past, to Okinawa or Paleolithic times—look anywhere. Scary and strange as sticking with a limited number of meals might seem now that we're bombarded with self-interested messages to the contrary, *your* ancestors did it. And not just your distant ancestors, but until quite recently. There is abundant, overwhelming precedent for this behavior, all over the place, and near at hand. You can do it, too.

Here are some numbers to back up the cross-cultural association between snacking and obesity: In America we now get 26 percent of our total calories from snacks—twice the amount as in 1976—and our obesity rate is now over 30 percent. The French get only 8 percent of their calories from snacks, and their obesity rate is correspondingly lower at 11 percent. The Chinese get less than 1 percent of their calories from snacks, and their obesity rate is a mere 3 percent.[3] Anyplace you look where statistics like this are available you'll see the same pattern: More snacking means more obesity.

Do the French Really Eat Like This?

> *The French [in this study] ate less than one snack a day. Here in the United States, we have about three snacks a day.*
>
> —R. Curtis Ellison, M.D., professor of
> preventive medicine and epidemiology
> at Boston University[4]

 Snacking is simply not part of the culture.

—Annie Jacquet-Bentley,
Parisian restaurant consultant[5]

Sadly, the culture seems to be changing. "Le snacking" (it's such a foreign concept to the French that they had to borrow our word!) and obesity are on the rise: "In France, as in much of the world, the culprit is changing eating habits, experts said, as France's powerful culture of traditional meals has given way to the pressures of modern life. The French now eat fewer formal meals than they did just a decade ago and they snack more."[6]

✱ It used to be impossible to find food outside of meal times. Now home refrigerators are full of it.

—Dr. France Bellisle,
Centre National de Recherche Scientifique[7]

How About the Chinese?

"Snacking is inconsequential in China, comprising only 0.9 percent of energy intake....Chinese children are less overweight, less inactive, and less likely to ingest calories as snacks than children in the United States."[8]

The Americans?

And then, of course, there's us: "Between 1977–78 and 2001–02, the percent of the U.S. population eating three or more snacks a day increased four-fold from 11 percent to 42 percent. In 2001–02, snacks contributed 26 percent of total calories."[9]

Making Excess Visible

Snacking makes self-deception easy; it doesn't just sound like *sneaking*, it facilitates it. Your excess is spread out over so many little increments that no one, including yourself, can ever point to you at one moment in time and say, "Hey, *right now* you're eating too much!" Except for the fact that you're fat, you can put on a very convincing charade.

And self-deception in regard to overeating is a big issue. Most of us wouldn't gorge ourselves the way we do if we couldn't at least put on a show of restraint, even if only for ourselves.

When you stick with three single-plate meals, you can rely on your eyes again to spot excess. Excess becomes visible, unavoidably visible. You don't have to count, you can see it; in fact, it's difficult *not* to see it. Excess doesn't need to be smoked out of caves and tunnels; it volunteers itself. This is hugely important, not just because it makes monitoring easier but because it makes self-deception hard.

Why Is Everyone Else So Pro-Snack?

It may seem strange, given the striking contribution of snacking to our increased caloric intake since the 1970s, that all the messages you hear about it are so positive. But the reason for this is simple: Follow the money. You can't sell "no snacks." Snacks, on the other hand, especially the booming "healthy" snack segment, are a multi-billion-dollar industry. Fat people like to snack—that's why they're fat—so they're glad to hear pro-snack talk. Avarice + gluttony (and a little bit of sloth) = obesity.

Why Do People Snack So Much More Than They Used To?

Cheap, convenient snack foods are abundant today; this is something very new, historically. We've got no natural defenses against them. These snack foods give us the option to never be hungry, even for a moment, so why not take it? And once you are accustomed to permasnacking the slightest bit of hunger seems like something awful, irresistible, and unnatural. Plus there are people who make a lot of money from snack foods, whether healthy or unhealthy. There isn't anyone who makes money from the absence of snack foods. So the messages are very one-sided.

Cutler, in the article cited earlier, argues that simple economics—the cheapness of snack foods made possible by recent technological advances—was sufficient in itself to explain the dramatic rise in snacking. These technologies tend to originate in America and then spread out to the rest of the world, just like the rising obesity rates they seem to be causing.

Other researchers cite the influence of TV:

The prevalence of eating snacks while watching television increases with age, and is associated with an increase in energy intake and decreased fruit and vegetable consumption. Research on the influence of food advertising shows that advertising during the time that early adolescents typically watch television is predominately for micronutrient-poor energy-dense foods, and the time spent watching television is linked to adolescents' consumption of these foods, including higher intakes of energy, fat, sweet and salty snacks, and carbonated beverages.[10]

And apparently it works both ways:

The coexistence of snacking behavior may also be likely to be cued by either television viewing and/or the snack (particularly after school) and be a prompt to switch on the television. If this is the case, then interventions targeting snacking behavior, rather than television viewing, may be more successful in reducing both caloric intake and time spent viewing television.[11]

So a great side benefit of no snacks is that it might cut down on the time you waste watching TV.

I think the most interesting factor in the rise of snacking is the decline and fall of the home-cooked family meal. When women entered the workforce in significant numbers, it was a great gain for them and for society as a whole; but, like everything, it also had a cost. There was no longer, in most homes, a dedicated cook and meal enforcer. Meals became less regular, less sacred. Snacks filled the gaps.

I'm not suggesting we turn back the clock and keep mom at home in the kitchen. I'm just suggesting we realize that there ain't no such thing as a free lunch (or snack). We have to acknowledge the costs of our trade-offs, that these costs can be real and damaging even if the greater good for which they were done was worth it, and we have to take steps to minimize and repair that damage. When unconscious social structures that keep us eating well fall away, we have to replace them with conscious ones; ones that, like the No S Diet, resemble the old structures that worked so well.

I don't know how important it is for us as individuals who are trying to lose weight to choose between these theories. The problem—frequent snacking—is clear, and so is the solution—reduced snacking (no snacking except on S days). Speculating about the ultimate cause of the snacking epidemic may be interesting, but it's not necessary. I like the last theory best (the decline of the home-cooked meal), not because it's the best supported by the evidence (that would have to go to the simple economics theory) but because, by putting the emphasis on traditional family meals, it makes our efforts seem more positive. There are, after all, other benefits to a home-cooked meal shared with family and friends that go beyond mere energy intake.

Aren't Snacks Metabolized More Efficiently Than Meals?

Under laboratory conditions, some studies have suggested that people who eat a controlled amount of calories over the course of many small meals burn them off slightly more efficiently than people who eat the same amount of calories in the traditional three meals a day. This is the principle behind books like *The 3 Hour Diet*.[12] But in the real world, people who snack wind up eating so many more calories that whatever metabolic boost they may derive from frequent eating is overwhelmed.

From a 2005 article published in the *International Journal of Obesity*:

> *Obese subjects were more frequent snackers than reference subjects and women were more frequent snackers than men. Snacks were positively related to energy intake, irrespective of physical activity. Sweet, fatty food groups were associated with snacking and contributed considerably to energy intake. Snacking needs to be considered in obesity treatment, prevention and general dietary recommendations.*[13]

The term *energy intake* makes it sound so positive; but they mean *calories*. From a 2002 article in *Medicina Clinica*:

> *Snacking was positively associated with a higher probability of gaining weight.... Our data suggest a direct association between snacking and weight gain in middle-aged people.*[14]

In fact, *occasional snacking* is probably the wrong term for the continuous, automatic eating most of us do nowadays. From a 2004 article in *Harvard Magazine*:

> *"The French explanation for why Americans are so big is simple,"* said Jody Adams, chef/partner of Rialto, a restaurant in Harvard Square, *"We eat lots of sugar, and we eat between meals. In France,*

no one gets so fat as to sue the restaurant!" Indeed,
the national response to our glut of comestibles is
apparently to eat only one meal all day long. We
eat everywhere and at all times: at work, at play,
and in transit.[15]

Even if you aren't one of these unconscious perma-snackers, but deliberately graze in order to overclock your metabolism, snacking still isn't a good idea. The problem with such grazing is that it's impossible to get a sense of how much you are eating without paying an exorbitant amount of attention, counting calories, points, and so on. Doing all that math is way too much conscious effort to sustain for the long term, and it's not something you can automate into unconscious habit. It's *too much* mental work to do consciously, and the *wrong kind* of mental work to do unconsciously.

Stick with single-plate meals, and you get a shortcut to measuring how much you are eating that is accurate enough to be useful but unobtrusive enough to be sustainable. You don't need to count; you can eyeball how much you're eating. And after a while, you barely have to do that because it becomes habitual. Counting, arithmetic, is never going to become an unconscious habit.

What About Healthy Snacks?

I've been focusing on packaged snack foods here, but even healthy snacks are a problem. Partially in themselves, because they have some calories and you're not effectively monitoring them, but more importantly because by eating them outside the context of a meal

✳ Don't let the complicated *perfect* be the enemy of the simple *good enough*.

you're effectively justifying their exclusion from your meals—and their replacement with less healthy, more caloric stuff. Psychologically, getting your healthy fix before a meal means you think you can skip it during the meal. You'll think, "I ate my vegetables already, I'm not going to blow a significant part of my meal on salad. I'm going to max out on fatty, carby, supercaloric stuff!"

And remember, when you snack on any kind of food, healthy as it may be in itself, nothing is ever "in itself," and habit gets confused. Your internal metronome gets upset. Your meal–meal–meal pattern has been disrupted, and you're more likely to snack again. And your healthy snack today may not be so healthy tomorrow. If you really could limit yourself to raw carrot sticks, it wouldn't be so bad (maybe), but don't kid yourself: You probably can't. The healthy snack is like a bribe to your conscience from your appetite for future unhealthy snacks, a token virtue that's just a pretext for vice, a credit for future debits.

Want to eat healthy food? Then eat healthy meals. If you know you have just three, you'll make them count. I'm perfectly aware that an orange between meals is not going kill you, that, taken in itself, it's perfectly healthy. But the idea is to have the orange instead of, not in addition to and in justification of, some unhealthy part of your meal. The problem is primarily one of self-discipline, and if you start making all kinds of exceptions, you'll fail.

Habit is like a wild animal: powerful, but dumb. You have to keep your desired behaviors nice and simple if you want habit to work for you. "Healthy snacks" is too complicated for wild-animal habit to understand, and healthy meals provide sufficient opportunity to eat healthy food. Don't let the complicated *perfect* be the enemy of the simple *good enough*.

What About Diet Bars?

Any diet that sells a bar or a snack food is a total scam. I'd rather eat a Snickers bar than a diet bar, because at least then I'd be psychologically budgeting for it. Diet bars should be called "self-deception bars." They legitimate the bad habit of snacking, indulge your self-destructive gluttony, and line the pockets of the enabling diet guru. In case you're wondering why most other diet gurus are so pro-snack, *this is it*. The diet bar is what separates the total scams from the mere fads.

Snacking Is Bad for Your Teeth!

You probably already know that sugar is bad for your teeth. That's so obvious I won't even bother going into it in the next chapter. But did you know that *snacking* also increases your risk for tooth decay? According to the American Dental Association:

> Not only what you eat but when you eat makes a
> big difference in your dental health. Eat a balanced

diet and limit between-meal snacks....Foods that
are eaten as part of a meal cause less harm. More
saliva is released during a meal, which helps wash
foods from the mouth and helps lessen the effects
of acids.[16]

I find this interesting not just in itself, but as an additional sign that snacking is not, as our contemporary conventional wisdom would have it, a necessary and normal behavior, but something strange and unprecedented that our bodies are not quite equipped to handle.

What If I Get Hungry Between Meals?

The solution to hunger between meals is this: Prepare big enough meals + build the habit of "mealing" + reach for a beverage if you get too hungry or to preempt hunger if you know it is going to be a problem. It really does get better, especially as the habit component of the equation grows.

Try drinking a beverage before you get hungry. Thirst is often confused with hunger. I know this is hard to believe when you're in the throes of it, but by drinking proactively you might preempt such "hunger" and not even have to believe. Although noncaloric drinks are obviously preferable, it is technically okay to reach for a caloric drink (as long as it isn't loaded with sugar) if you think that's what it will take to see you through to your next meal without snacking on solid food (see page 54 for more guidance on this issue).

Although you shouldn't be miserable, the idea that hunger is somehow wrong is a novel and misguided

✳ Try drinking a beverage before you get hungry. Thirst is often confused with hunger.

concept. Hunger isn't a disease. It's natural and good to be hungry before a meal. Not for hours and not painfully, but habit and attitude can go a long way toward mitigating that.

Good, regular habits (and full meals) will make hunger more bearable, even pleasant. The old adage that "appetite is the best sauce" isn't just irritating moralizing, it's true—I've experienced it. If this seems inconceivable to you now, it's only because you're in the thrall of some very unnatural habits. With the No S Diet, you'll quickly build good habits, and this will seem like the most normal thing in the world. You'll be surprised when you see people eating between meals. You'll think, as your mom used to tell you, that they're spoiling their appetites.

Isn't It Better to Eat When I'm Hungry?

You often hear formulas like "Eat only when you're hungry" and "Eat what you want, not what you should" touted as liberating, antidiet weight-loss wisdom. But despite their appeal to nature and their warm-and-fuzzy feel, these formulas are no more effective than "Don't eat too much." In fact, they're worse. They are not merely impossible advice, they are *bad* advice. And they are profoundly *un*natural.

I have two cats. The concept of *should* is utterly alien to them. But if I give them too much food, they happily eat it and get fat. They want too much. So do I. Superabundance is not a natural problem, so we don't have good instincts to deal with it. Why would we? No animal (until us, now, perhaps) ever died because there was too much food. Plenty died because there was too little. That all too common scenario is the reason the feeling of hunger evolved—to avoid starvation. So it's not going to be a very reliable guide to moderating intake; that's just not its job.

Eating whenever you're hungry is not only unnatural, it's uncivilized. Human beings in traditional societies didn't eat when they were hungry; food was too scarce and precious and hard to prepare for that. Our ancestors were hungry *a lot*. When times were good, they ate at regular, discrete, social meals, with real gratitude. When times were not so good, they experienced something that makes our "hunger" look like a joke.

Furthermore, if you're a so-called emotional eater, you may not get an honest answer to, "Am I really hungry?" Depression is going to attempt to pass itself off as hunger. So will stress. So will countless other emotions. And they'll be quite convincing.

It's harder to deceive yourself when the question is, "Is it mealtime?" or "Is this a brownie and is it 4 a.m. Monday morning?" Self-deception is a powerful force, and you can't afford to be naive about it. *No snacks* blocks this kind of self-deception. It simply doesn't matter when you're hungry; you're not allowed to eat.

Real or imagined hunger is not a valid excuse. And soon enough, if you're firm, you'll stop even trying to make emotional excuses; any real hunger you have will start to coincide with mealtimes.

Although dieting may not have done much good for the problem of obesity, I don't think it's quite fair to say that it caused it. There is nothing new about rules governing the way people eat. What is new is that formerly the rules were externally imposed: by scarcity, by social structures, by tradition. When these external forces passed away, it was only to be expected that people would seek new rules. But most of those new rules were poorly thought out; they didn't resemble or even take into account the old rules that had served so well for thousands of generations.

I'm not saying we have no "nature" to work with in regard to eating, simply that it's not enough to rely on. Eating discrete meals is satisfying and natural; but without either social pressure, natural scarcity, rules, or habit, that natural satisfaction by itself isn't going to be enough to make you do it. It's just a foundation. You can and should work with it (as the No S Diet does), but don't expect it to do the work for you.

The sad thing about snacking to manage hunger is that *it doesn't even work*. "Research shows that after snacking, people are inclined to eat just as much at meals as they do when they don't snack," says David Levitsky.[17] We don't, outside of a lab, compensate for snack calories at mealtime—at all. By snacking, we just eat more. And no matter how efficient our metabolisms, we aren't going to be able to turn those extra calories into negative calories.

So don't eat when you're hungry. Don't eat when you're depressed. Don't eat when you've seen a good number on the scale and you think you can afford a few extra calories. Eat when it's *time* to eat, just like thin people did for thousands of years.

This doesn't mean you'll be starving all the time. Limit your intake to meals and your appetite will gradually learn that that's the time to get hungry.

What If I'm Not Hungry at Mealtime?

If you're not hungry at mealtime, you will be hungry an hour later, so eat preemptively. Once you get a regular routine of mealtime eating down, this won't happen much. Remember: You're the boss. You're the trainer. Your appetite is a dumb brute, an animal. You tell it when to get hungry; and, like Pavlov's dogs, it'll learn. If you let your appetite lead you, that's like the dog leading the trainer: not only counterproductive but degrading.

Is It Extra-Good to Eat Fewer Meals?

Skipping meals, especially breakfast, is strongly associated with obesity. It isn't extra-good—it's extra-bad. You may feel like you're doing something virtuous by depriving yourself of a meal, but in all likelihood, the calories you cut out now will come back later—with interest.

Remember that generations of people stayed thin on three meals a day. According to the USDA data cited earlier, the average number of calories ingested at dinner

---

✳ Meals are not the problem; they are the solution.

---

actually has *declined* since 1977.[18] It's snacks that are pumping all these extra calories into us. Meals are not the problem; they are the solution.

But a meal isn't just a meal. It's not just "one time." It's a link in the chain of habit. Skip a meal, and you are breaking the chain for the sake of a few less calories. That's just not worth it.

So no more than three meals but no less! Let the maximum be the minimum.

Do Drinks Count as Snacks?

The No S Diet does not count drinks (even caloric ones) as snacks. You can drink whenever you want, unless its something full of sugar, in which case it counts as a sweet (see Chapter 3). If you think you'll pop unless you get your pop, have a look at my hierarchy of soda alternatives (on page 56).

I don't count alcoholic beverages as S's, either. I usually have a drink or two a day, which is supposed to be very healthy. Two drinks is my "glass ceiling," however, because I've read (and experienced) that more than that can be pretty awful. If you have two drinks or less, I don't imagine they'll have much impact from a caloric point of view. If you drink much more, you may have a different sort of problem altogether.

The subject of drinks isn't to be viewed in purely negative terms. It's not just about avoiding liquid calories. Drink water proactively to ward off hunger. As I said earlier, thirst is often confused with hunger, and a glass of water can be an effective snack replacement. No, it doesn't taste quite as good, but yes it can do the trick.

Caloric drinks (as long as they're not full of sugar) are also acceptable snack substitutes. While liquid calories are qualitatively no different from solid-food calories, by reaching for a drink instead of a solid snack, the habit of not eating solid food between meals is still preserved, and you are unlikely to drink nonsugar drinks in sufficient quantities for it to be much of an issue, calorically speaking. So while noncaloric drinks between meals are preferable, if you're about to break down and start snacking, it's okay to have a glass of milk instead.

Whole milk is loaded with fat and calories. But guess how much whole milk Americans drank in the thin 1970s compared with Americans today? According to the USDA,[19] over three times *more* (25 gallons per person per year in 1970, but only 8 gallons today). In the even thinner 1940s, we drank almost six times more (45 gallons in 1945). All that skim and reduced-fat milk we now drink instead hasn't slimmed us down any (15 gallons today versus 6 gallons in 1970 and 4 gallons in 1945). It has probably only lubricated our consciences to make us ignore all the sugar soda we're drinking (22 gallons in 1970 compared to 56 gallons today).[20] Dairy is actually the only top-level category of food substance tracked by the USDA's Economic Research Service to have shown a *decrease* in calorie consumption since 1970.[21]

Whole milk, like 100 percent fruit juice, is very

filling. It's difficult to drink large quantities at once because you can taste the fat and calories. You can get away with drinking a much smaller amount, without the false sense of security that lower-calorie milk products give you. It also tastes much better. So although it isn't a technical requirement of the No S Diet, I would recommend sticking with whole milk rather than skim or reduced-fat milk. Our bodies have evolved to expect milk to be fatty and caloric, and the statistics show that tricking our bodies with less fatty substitutes has clearly not worked as a weight loss strategy—quite the contrary.

A Hierarchy of Soft-Drink Alternatives

Pop isn't just pop. Psychologically, it's a lot more to many people. It's a break, a ritual, and a drug like cigarettes. So we need to find you a surrogate, something to take its place.

Any potential replacement needs to be evaluated for three factors:

* Health impact
* Ritual
* Drug appeal

Water has a positive effect on our health, not much ritual, and no drug appeal. Cigarettes are wonderful for ritual and drug appeal but have a nasty tendency to kill you. Tea and coffee (easy on the sugar and cream; I drink mine black) do pretty well in every department. If that's not up your alley, diet drinks are probably better than nondiet drinks, except (1) I'm suspicious about what the awful chemicals in those products are going to do to you down the road and (2) the sweetness messes with the habit-forming portion of your brain (you stay addicted to the taste).

So from best to worst, here are my suggestions:

* Water
* Tea (green, especially)
* Coffee (black, especially)
* Milk (whole isn't so bad; see page 55)
* 100 percent fruit juice (see page 77)
* Diet soda
* Sugar soda

Get as close to the top of this list as you can. If diet soda is the best you can do right now, don't beat yourself up about it. Revisit the issue in a couple of months when you've graduated to a higher level of willpower.

Does It Matter When I Eat My Meals?

Technically, you can eat your meals whenever you'd like on the No S Diet, but it will be harder to form habits unless you keep more or less regular times. Habit is like music; regular rhythm and tempo make it easier to carry a tune—or a behavior.

It's also important to space your meals out so you don't get too hungry. For me, that means breakfast at 7:30, lunch at 1:00, dinner at 6:30. I'm not religious about this, but it's usually what I do, and I think a morning–afternoon–evening schedule is helpful.

Statistically, people tend to snack most in the afternoons. So pay particular attention to the gap between lunch and dinner. Eat a large lunch, preferably not too early. Make sure you have a beverage or some chewing gum on hand to resort to if you find yourself getting too hungry.

What If My Doctor Says I Need to Eat More Than Three Meals a Day?

If you have a medical condition that requires you to eat more often, you can still do so and be a proud No S Dieter. Just make sure to figure out what number of meals is right for you, stick with it (no changing the magic number every day!), and invest in some really small plates. And talk to your doctor, of course. As for the rest of you, pretend you never read this. It's for people with doctor's notes only.

There are cultures that had an official fourth meal, so there is precedent for this. But I think it's a relic from back in the days when people burned thousands of calories a day doing strenuous work in the fields. Given the baseline of excess with which most people come into the No S Diet, you should still be able to lose weight with four meals a day, but there is more opportunity for abuse, and even in the best-case scenario it will be slow. Regular three-meal No S Diet weight loss is slow enough for most people. I wouldn't try more than that unless you have a good medical reason (or the patience of Job).

What If I Have a Crazy Schedule?

Some people, for reasons beyond their immediate control, find themselves faced with unacceptably long gaps between meals. This might be because they have to work a double shift, or carry a heavy college course load, or have to coordinate meals with a spouse who has a very different schedule.

Short term, if you have a schedule like this, consider adding a fourth mini-meal. It's not ideal, but it's better than unscheduled snacking, and it may be the best thing you can do under the circumstances.

Long term, the best thing to do is try to change your circumstances and get yourself on a less crazy schedule. I know it may not be easy to make such sweeping changes, but regularity is *that* important. It's worth the investment. Eating and sleeping are fundamental routines, your most basic internal metronome. If you can't get regularity in them, it's going to be difficult to build any other kind of regular habits.

But Thin People Sometimes Snack

There are people who can get up in the morning without an alarm clock. I'm not one of them. There are also people who have an instinctive sense of moderation when it comes to eating. If you're reading this book, I assume you're not one of them. Others might be able to snack without eating to excess, but you need clear rules: the dietary equivalent of an alarm clock. And I think that if you carefully observed the overall snacking behavior of most thin people, it would be closer to

"no snacks" than to the permasnacking of most overweight people. Their instinctive perfect isn't replicable,
so you're going to have to settle for the explicit good
enough of the No S Diet. And it's really not such a bad
good enough.

The media often hold up the traditional French diet
as exemplary, and I've made reference to it myself. As
I've mentioned, French people don't snack as much or
eat as many sweets as overweight Americans do. But
their behavior obviously doesn't conform 100 percent
to the rules of the No S Diet. They sometimes snack
(and not just on S days!). They sometimes eat sweets
during the week. So why can't we? Well, the problem
is that it is very hard to precisely replicate complex eating behaviors like this. And even French people would
have trouble eating like French people outside the discipline and support structure of French society (which,
by the way, is becoming less and less supportive all the
time). The No S Diet is a useful approximation of traditional eating structures, not an exact replica. We can't
build an exact replica without rebuilding a whole society. That's not possible, and it's not necessary for solving the problem at hand. The No S Diet rules are close
enough—and good enough—to solve this problem and
are far, far simpler to adhere to.

3

No Sweets

A Saner Form of Low Carb

The average American consumes more than 100 pounds
of sugar a year, well over 10 times the average amount
consumed in colonial days.[1] This is so obviously excessive that I'm a little baffled that diet gurus have seen the
need to probe more deeply for invisible culprits for the
obesity epidemic, such as carbs in general. In their inves-
tigative zeal, the gurus have managed to get everyone
all excited about these dietary bogeymen hiding in our
midst. What they have *not* managed to do is get us any
thinner. The current incarnation of the low-carb craze
started almost 10 years ago (after previously becoming
popular in the 1960s and before that in the 1860s), yet

we're fatter now than we've ever been before in human history.

The problem is not dietary enemies that we can't see. The problem is that we don't open our eyes to see the enemy right in front of our faces. Sugar is a carb, too, after all. But unlike other carbohydrates, sugar is easy to detect; we don't need charts and tables; our taste buds are sufficient. And while scientists are still arguing about whether or not, and to what degree, carbs are actually vital for your health, sugar is obviously, indisputably bad for you, beyond a very small amount. No scientist, doctor, or dentist on earth thinks added sugar is good for you. There is no medical disagreement about whether drastically reducing our sugar intake would benefit most people.

And the degree of our excess is so great that we wouldn't even have to cut out sugar entirely to see enormous benefits. We wouldn't have to sacrifice any pleasure worth mentioning. We could enjoy twice as much sugar as our relatively recent ancestors did, even five times as much, and still be in better shape than we are now. So why expand the problem to carbs, a bigger, more difficult, more ambiguous problem, when there is so much obvious excess, easily detectable and indisputably harmful excess, here at the sugar level? Sugar is the low-hanging fruit, the easy part of the carb problem—and it's enough of a problem, together with the other issues addressed by the No S Diet, to make a decisive difference. In a way, it's a shortcut to low-carb eating, bypassing the tedium of constantly having to consult a manual, bypassing the sense of deprivation of having to go without so many different foods, and

bypassing the medical risk of a historically unprecedented and medically controversial behavior.

The reason hidden culprits like carbs are such an
attractive enemy is simple: our guilty consciences. An
obvious foe would make us accomplices, not innocent
victims. After all, we *know* we eat too much sugar; it's
right there in front of us. We can't blame the junk-food
companies and other evildoers for somehow tricking
us into getting fat. We have to take responsibility; we
have to admit that we did something obviously wrong.
That's hard to do and unpleasant to believe, so we keep
going back to diet plans that deceive us and work us up
into states of righteous indignation against nefarious
outside forces.

All too often, we'd rather think of ourselves as powerless dupes than own up to our bad decisions. I did this
myself, but in retrospect I find it baffling. Apart from its
mere inefficacy, apart from being just dumb, it is actually
a terrible and degrading way of looking at oneself. On
the surface, it seems as if you were being kind to yourself, letting yourself off the hook. But it flatters only
the worst part of yourself and completely casts off the
best. A sense of responsibility is a powerful, ennobling
thing. To cast that off for the sake of indulging gluttony is even worse than the gluttony itself.

With sugar, we can't make such excuses. Our excessive
sugar intake is obviously problematic—on three levels: It
is obviously *too much* (the quantities involved are unprecedented and enormous), it is obviously *detectable* (we
have a whole sensory apparatus specifically dedicated to
detecting sweetness), and it is obviously *bad for you* (not
even the deep pockets of the sugar lobby have managed

to buy any medically favorable research). You can't miss this problem. It's a target as big as a house—a gaudily painted house. The problem isn't its mystery; the problem is its magnitude. I hope I've convinced you that sugar is a sufficiently serious problem to be worth focusing on. Now I'm going to try to convince you of the opposite: that it's also a tractable problem, one that's not so serious or irreversible that you should feel overwhelmed by it.

Toppling the House of Sugar

The *no sweets* rule makes the excessive sugar problem manageable. It does this in two subtle but powerful ways: clarity and moderation.

First off, note that the rule is *no sweets* rather than *no sugar*. This is an important distinction. Sweets are foods and drinks that *clearly* contain a lot of added sugar: cookies, cake, sugar soda, Pop-Tarts, ice cream, Cap'n Crunch cereal. Foods that contain some sugar but aren't primarily composed of it are okay. You don't have to make yourself and everyone around you crazy by checking lists of ingredients; your taste buds will let you know. And your sweet tooth won't suffer total deprivation. You can still enjoy foods that contain *some* sugar: fresh fruit, coffee with a teaspoon or two, the coating on your pan-seared salmon. Most foods are either clearly okay or clearly not okay. And if you have to wonder—as with slightly sweet foods such as yogurt, peanut butter, adult breakfast cereal, ketchup—it's probably fine. The really egregious offenders represent such a large part of the problem that they're all you need to worry about. Considering how much sugar we

✱ The chocolate chip cookie that might otherwise have tripped you up is now an incentive to get you through to the weekend, when you can legitimately enjoy it.

normally eat, just cutting that amount in half will make a huge difference. This rule easily does that and more.

No sweets is not overambitious. It's firm, but *moderate*. It limits itself to just the excessive part of our sugar consumption and gives a wide berth to our sweet tooth's legitimate (and, frankly, irresistible) claims. Sugar isn't evil, nor is our enjoyment of it; it's the excess that is bad. With this rule, our enormous appetite for sweet is given some wiggle room, it doesn't feel mortally threatened. No sweets is a stick, as in the proverbial carrot and stick, not a guillotine.

And the No S Diet provides a carrot to go with this stick: On weekends and holidays (S days) your sweet tooth is rewarded for its compliance during the week. S days aren't just a mere concession to overwhelming appetite, they're a way of conscripting the power of this appetite to work for you, as a motivating force. Instead of sabotaging your efforts by being a constant temptation, your appetite for sweets will sustain them, as an incentive. So now instead of fighting against this wild-animal appetite, you've tamed and harnessed it to pull you along. The chocolate chip cookie that might otherwise have tripped you up is now an incentive to get you through to the weekend, when you can legitimately enjoy it.

How Much Sugar Do Americans Eat?

According to a report by the Economic Research Service (ERS) of the U.S. Department of Agriculture (USDA), the average American ingested 105 pounds of added sugar in 2001. That's about 20 percent of the total calories consumed. You could make a snowman out of that. It means most of us eat our body weight in sugar every two years. And this is a pretty conservative number. The ERS assumes that more than 40 pounds of "delivered" sugar is "lost" (that is, thrown out), which I find a little hard to believe, but I guess we're wastrels as well as gluttons.[2]

How do you think that compares with the sugar intake of our ancestors? We don't have to look at hunter-gatherer societies to find a striking contrast or even to the times before Columbus, when consumption was close to nil because there was no refined sugar in most places. Let's take 1821, when it was 10 pounds (that's delivered, not ingested!).[3]

And we can get closer still:

Since the 1970s, there has been a 35 percent increase in the calories Americans consume from sugar added to their foods by the food industry. More comes from soft drinks than from any other food category, even desserts.[4]

It doesn't take an Atkins zealot to see there's a problem here. Indeed, why bother taking it to the next level by severely restricting carbs in general, with all the potential health issues that raises, when there is so much of a problem at the sugar level alone?

How Is *No Sweets* Different from *No Sugar*?

I've discussed this already, but it bears repeating: By *sweets* I mean something in which the principal source of calories is added sugar, something that actually tastes sweet. You don't have to go checking lists of ingredients and driving waiters crazy; your taste buds will let you know. Foods with some sugar are fine. A good rule of thumb is, "Is it sweet enough to be a dessert?"

Sugar is not inherently evil. It gives real pleasure, and that's worth something. Sacrificing that pleasure completely isn't virtuous, and it isn't even helpful. "No sweets, except on S days" balances the pleasure of sugar against its cost. It goes further: It uses that pleasure for a net benefit.

Is No Sweets Enough?

The rule *no sweets* is enough to make a decisive difference in terms of your total caloric intake. Although it is true that many processed foods contain a surprising amount of sugar, this pales in comparison to the amount of sugar consumed through unambiguously sweet foods. Given the quantities of these foods that we eat, it would be amazing if we weren't fat. The frequently asked questions (FAQs) section of the Unilever ice cream website boasts, "The average American eats around 45 pints (5.63 gallons) of ice cream a year, more than any other nationality."[5] According to the Center for Science in the Public Interest, adolescents get 13 percent of their daily calories from soft drinks.[6] Per capita soft drink consumption has increased almost 500 percent over the past 50 years to become the single biggest source of calories in the American diet. Cut out these egregious sugary excesses during the week and you will cut out plenty.[7]

Is No Sweets Too Much?

On to the opposite concern! Some people worry that they will feel deprived by giving up sweets during the week. And in the very beginning, that might be true. But, ultimately, I think you'll come to enjoy sweets even more on the No S Diet than you ever did before.

First off, keep in mind that you can still enjoy foods that contain some sugar during the week. It's far from complete deprivation.

But, more importantly, the sweets you can legitimately enjoy on S days will taste better than they ever did before. This isn't just because you can enjoy them with a clear conscience or because of the anticipation that's been building up during the week. It's also because your sweets won't just *seem* better, they'll *be* better. Why? Because limited opportunity will push you to take best advantage of it. When you have only a weekend or a holiday in which to indulge, you have to be choosy about what you indulge in: You'll buy or make something better than you would have otherwise. Instead of mindlessly snacking on cheap junk in front of the television, you'll treat yourself to something really special. By limiting quantity, you improve quality.

I'm not some food-hating, pleasure-begrudging voice in the wilderness. I'm not telling you to give up sweets

*   By limiting quantity, you improve quality.

completely. I love sweets. But I love them even more on
S days. That way I can love them unreservedly, without
also hating them for what they do to my body. On S
days, I make sure to pick out something really nice, to
make it count. Sweets weren't designed for daily, routine consumption, physically or spiritually. Deserve
your desserts. They taste much better that way.

Why Not No Starch?

Starch starts with S, and it's a very unpopular substance with many dieters nowadays. But the No S Diet
does not restrict it. Why?

For one thing, the *no sweets* restriction is sufficient;
if you add more restrictions you don't really gain anything and you risk overburdening yourself. That's reason enough, as far as I'm concerned. But there's also the
issue that *no starch* isn't as clear as *no sweets*. Starch
doesn't have a striking taste. So you'll have to rely on
books and tables instead of your taste buds to identify
which foods to avoid.

Another complicating factor is that you clearly do
need some starch. An absolute prohibition would be
dangerous, and it's very unclear where you should draw
the line. Last, the jury is still out one whether or not
an extremely low-starch/low-carb diet is medically safe.
Why take risks when *no sweets* will do the job?

What is starch, anyway? I'm amazed at how many people who claim to be avoiding it don't even know. It's one of three kinds of dietary carbohydrates—the others are sugar and fiber. Starch is not some Frankenstein ingredient out of a pharmaceutical lab but is found abundantly in natural foods such as grains, roots, tubers, fruits, and seeds. It's so abundant in our food supply that, since the dawn of agriculture at least, it has been the chief source of our caloric intake.[8]

Yes, that's right, historically, most of the calories people have consumed since they learned to grow plants were from carbohydrates, and from starch specifically. And, historically, most people were thin. Without starch, they would have been dead. It seems odd to target a substance that kept our ancestors alive and thin for thousands of years as the culprit for the recent obesity epidemic. With the unprecedented amounts of meat and fat that we in our rich society today can enjoy, we're *already* eating low-carb, as a percentage of total calories, compared to our poorer ancestors (and neighbors). So why do something totally historically unprecedented, when we have thousands of years of evidence, from *billions* of people, that eating a much higher percentage of carbs (and starch) than we currently do will not, in itself, make us fat?

What people historically did not eat a lot of is sugar. That is the really striking *substantive* difference between our diet and that of our skinny ancestors. Yes, they managed to find some sugar (or, more likely, honey), and prized it highly. But it was rare, expensive, a festive treat; precisely what the No S Diet aims to make it again.

If the past will not persuade you, consider the future.

If more and more people really were to start eating low-carb, and get more and more of their calories from animal protein, the environmental consequences would be devastating. According to a United Nations report quoted in the *New York Times*, already "global livestock grazing and feed production use '30 percent of the land surface of the planet,'" and "livestock are responsible for about 18 percent of the global warming effect"—more than cars, airplanes, and all forms of transportation *combined*.[9] Worried about everyone in currently skinny, high-carb India and China getting cars like us and what that will do to the environment? Worry, too, about them going Atkins, even just halfway.

The truth is, we fat Westerners *already* eat a low-carb diet. Compared to people in other parts of the world and to our own ancestors, we get a much higher percentage or our calories from fat and protein than from carbohydrates. Ever heard that old saw about "all the rice in China"? Well, that's what they eat, mostly. It's their chief source of calories. And it's white rice. No one in Asia, except perhaps a few Western expats, eats brown rice. Ditto in India. Not especially fat countries. And that's about half the world's population right there. The simple fact is that people in most parts of the word can't afford to eat as much meat and fat as we do today; and until recently, we couldn't afford it either.

Does Fake Sugar Count as a Sweet?

I would avoid fake sugar products for three reasons.

First, they tend to be pretty disgusting. Second, you

know that in 10 years scientists are going to discover that they're even worse for you than real sugar. And, finally, you might be fooling your taste buds, but you're also fooling the habit-forming portion of your brain that's supposed to be learning to live with fewer sweets. It's bad psychology, and the whole premise of the No S Diet is that psychology is the most essential component of weight loss. As a member of the No S Diet bulletin board put it, you are training "a poor and stupid part of the brain. Don't confuse it by thinking like a nutritionist. Think like a dog trainer."

So, do artificial sweeteners officially count as an S? No, not technically. But I'd be surprised if you could eat a lot of them without reverting to genuine sugar. Consider the fact that despite (or perhaps because of) the proliferation of sugar substitutes in recent decades, consumption of actual sugar has still gone up. People seem to be eating artificial sweeteners *in addition to*, not instead of real sugar. They probably feel so virtuous for eating this artificial stuff that they think they can afford to indulge in more real guilt.

Naturally slim people do not cram themselves with diet products. Neither should you. Save your sweets for S days, when you can *really* enjoy them, in their unadulterated form. It's so much less risky in terms of habit building and so much better in terms of taste. By sticking with real sugar, you'll enjoy it more and wind up eating far less. You'll know what you're dealing with and won't feel the false sense of security and entitlement that comes from food substitutes.

Besides the statistical likelihood of your reverting to the real thing anyway, the idea of eating fake sugar and fake food in general has always seemed intrinsically awful to me. According to Greek mythology, the food in the underworld, Hades, looks beautiful and tempting; but when you bite into it, it tastes like dust. And then you have to stay in the underworld forever. Modern fake food has always seemed a little analogous to this to me, tricking the appetite with insubstantial, and perhaps dangerous, illusions. I've found the image of the dusty, damning food of Hades useful fortification in those rare moments when I've been tempted by simulacra.

Can I Put Sugar in My Coffee?

Go ahead and add sugar to your coffee. It's amazing how much people agonize over this calorically insignificant borderline case. Do you know how many spoonfuls of sugar you'd have to put in your coffee to match the sugar in one can of Coke? The answer is 10. (There are 39 grams of sugar in a can of Coca-Cola, and 4 grams of sugar in a teaspoon.) No one in the course of human history has ever put that many spoonfuls of sugar into his or her coffee, so relax. Enjoy your coffee. Your energies are much better directed elsewhere. (Do watch out for presweetened coffee drinks, though; those "desserts in a cup" can easily match the sugar content of a can of soda.)

So why do people tend to make such a big fuss over this? The quick answer is big profit margins and advertising budgets for sugar-substitute manufacturers. But the sugar lobby is pretty powerful, too, and pushes in the opposite direction. So I don't think that entirely explains it.

A bigger factor is that fussing over their coffee sweetener lets people put on a constant show of how virtuous they are. They get to assume a dainty look and ask, "Do you have any Sweet'N Low?" or "Do you have any Splenda?" (Subtext: "I might look fat, but see how virtuous I am!") They're pennywise and 250-pounds foolish. It sounds ridiculous because no one in their presence is fooled by such displays, but people do this all the time. To many people, a demonstration of virtue, no matter how unconvincing, is enough. Of course, the real purpose of this show is *self*-deception, allowing a fleeting sensation of virtue—a feeling almost as good as the real thing and much easier to come by. It's clear, with this behavior in mind, why gluttony used to be considered a moral vice: Because, as it's usually practiced, it's also dishonest.

With the No S Diet, there's no show. It's the opposite. Your excess is all out in the open. Instead of pretending to be virtuous in public and gorging in secret, you emphasize your vice (drawing attention to it with embarrassingly big plates, openly enjoying sweets on S days) and use shame to keep yourself in line. Honesty, shame, virtue: old-fashioned stuff, like being thin.

Do I Have to Start Checking Ingredients?

Don't worry about ingredient lists. If a food doesn't have enough sugar to taste very sweet, there's no problem. Furthermore, I wouldn't worry too much about borderline foods like yogurt or peanut butter and jelly sandwiches. If these are a problem for you—that is, if you eat them every day and lay it on thick—then make them foods you eat only on S days. If not, don't. Just by targeting the really egregious offenders, you'll be cutting out a lot of calories. And you'll be that much more likely to stick with the plan. If you're like most First Worlders, it's a little revolting to think about how much unambiguously lousy food you consume. So forget the borderline cases, the clear-cut cases are enough. Don't overburden yourself trying to do more.

Do Fruits Count as Sweets?

Fruits are not S foods; they're fine. Fruits are a big help, in fact, because they're the sweetest thing you can eat during the week; they'll take the edge off your sugar cravings. And without all that overstimulation of your sweet tooth, you'll enjoy them more than you ever did before.

Just make sure to enjoy them with your meals, of course, and not in between. Besides being tasty and healthy, fruit also tends to be bulky, so it crowds out less healthy stuff, which is a great help in keeping down the calorie count of even fully loaded single-plate meals.

What About Natural Sugars?

Are "natural" sweeteners like maple syrup, honey, and organic evaporated cane juice okay? Nope. Sorry. I don't care how well-marketed they are, they're sugar. Same rules apply as for the white stuff. Enjoy them straight-up on S days or as a minor ingredient in a larger dish during the week.

But Chocolate Is Good for You!

If you want to enjoy the newly discovered nutritional benefits of chocolate, be my guest—just make sure to consume it like the Aztecs did, without sugar (all of a sudden your interest in its supposed health benefits fades...), or reserve it for the weekends. Being fat because you eat too much chocolate is emphatically not good for you. And it's not just the chocolate in itself— by eating an unambiguous sweet, you are smudging a clear *no sweets* boundary, which will probably lead to further, nonchocolaty violations. It's amazing how up on the latest research people are when it comes to stuff they like to eat but know they really shouldn't.

For those of you just coming out of media seclusion, here's the deal about chocolate: A 2005 study reported in the *American Journal of Clinical Nutrition* indicated that eating 100 grams a day of dark chocolate for 15 days lowered blood pressure and improved the ability of the body to metabolize sugar.[10] But as Professor Graham MacGregor, chairman of the Blood Pressure Association, noted: "The benefits of eating chocolate are likely to be outweighed by the disadvantages as chocolate is high in sugar and fat."[11]

Another study, published in 2006 in the *Proceedings of the National Academy of Sciences*, attributed the low blood pressure and good cardiovascular health of the Kuna Indians, who live on the San Blas islands off the coast of Panama, to the large amounts of flavanol-rich cocoa they consume (three to four cups a day).[12] The problem? The Kuna's recipe requires fresh, hand-picked, high-flavanol cocoa beans. Flavanols make chocolate and cocoa taste bitter and so have been removed from most of the stuff you're likely to find in the supermarket. There is a world of difference between the fresh fruit they consume and the processed powder that makes it to us. It also requires massive quantities to see health benefits. A mere cup a day doesn't seem to do anything. Do you really want to drink *that* much hot cocoa every day? And don't put any milk in there; the proteins in milk seem to bind with the antioxidants in chocolate and block their effect.

I'm not completely joking about the Aztec hot chocolate. I've sworn not to fluff this book with recipes of any kind, but do a Google search for "Aztec hot chocolate" and you'll find plenty. The active ingredient (besides chocolate) is hot pepper. If you're really so concerned about the health benefits of chocolate, this is your drink—and it's No S approved. I haven't been able to find the Kuna recipe, but my suspicion is it's not very sweet either, or it would have been posted all over the place, with all the buzz it's gotten.

Do Sweet Drinks Count as Sweets?

If they're sweet enough, drinks count as sweets—and plenty are. Liquid form isn't an exemption. See page 54 for how unsweetened caloric drinks count as snacks (short answer: They don't).

Sugar soda and corn syrup "juice" drinks are a big deal, calorically speaking. Americans get an estimated 10 percent of their calories from such nutritionally bankrupt liquid carbohydrates; American kids get even more.[13]

I don't count 100 percent fruit juice as a sweet. Yes,

fruit juice is sweet. And it is very caloric. But it also tastes very caloric and almost syrupy. It's hard to drink the obscene quantities that we often do of similarly caloric but easier-going-down (and nutritionally worthless) soft drinks. I have yet to see someone drinking a 64-ounce Big Gulp of orange juice. And fruit juice is also very nutritious; it has a lot of calories, but they're not empty calories. To my mind, it's in an obviously different category than sugar soda. Honestly, if orange juice is really your problem, you don't have much of a problem.

If, despite this obvious difference, it turns out that fruit juice is enough of a problem for you, then by all means, count it as a sweet. But I don't think it will be, so don't preempt it; wait and see. The more restrictions you add, the greater the risk you'll just give up altogether.

Do note that I'm talking about *100 percent pure fruit juice* here. There are a lot of deceptively marketed fruit drinks that are mostly high-fructose corn syrup with a splash of fruit juice—stay away from those. If you really want to play it safe, squeeze your own. That way you're guaranteed to get pure, fresh, wholesome juice; and the labor involved will ensure both that you appreciate it and that don't drink too much. Besides being a lot of work, it's also eye-opening to see just how many oranges it takes to fill one modest glass; by the time you get to the second or third orange, shame at this excess will quench your thirst. Drink fruit juice and other caloric drinks out of fancy wine or martini glasses to make the smaller amounts seem like more and like something really special and dignified—and, like the alcoholic beverages you normally associate with such glasses, dangerous in large amounts.

4

No Seconds

A Shortcut to Portion Control

In most diets, measuring portion size involves consulting manuals or resorting to scales. How much does this piece of steak weigh? How many calories in an ounce of steak? What kind of steak is this exactly, and does it make a difference?

It's hard enough to stick to smaller portions; measuring them shouldn't be this hard. And it doesn't have to be. The no seconds rule of the No S Diet makes measuring portion size a snap. All you have to do is fit the food you'll eat in a meal on a single plate. No manuals, no scales—a *plate* is all the measuring equipment you need. It's not as precise as counting calories and weighing portions. But it's a heck of a lot easier, and

A *plate* is all the measuring equipment you need.

it's accurate *enough*. You're going to eat fewer calories each day; so what if you don't know the exact number?

Counting is too labor-intensive. It doesn't work. Almost no one is able to do it for more than a few months. So who cares if it's theoretically more accurate? You don't *need* that level of accuracy; you can't *sustain* that level of accuracy; and with the no seconds rule, you have a sufficiently accurate and infinitely more sustainable alternative.

So what exactly are we counting with no seconds? Seconds of what? Not "servings," whatever that means, but *plates*. The *no seconds* rule means you get one physical plate of food per meal. You can load up that plate with however much food you want—once. When you're done eating the food on that plate, the meal is over. No refills, and no eating again until your next meal.

Why use a crude measurement like plates instead of some more refined metric such as servings? Because the definition of one plate is clear (a plate may be large or small but it is clearly one, or clearly not), because an empty plate has strong psychological stopping power, because simple rules are easier to automate into unconscious habits, and because the evidence suggests (keep reading) that this crude metric is good enough to make a significant difference.

No seconds won't fix every instance of problematic portion control, but it will fix enough of them. You'll still eat some very large plates now and then; but if it's a few out of a hundred, or a few out of a thousand, who cares? With this simple rule, your long-term *average* calorie consumption per meal will, relatively painlessly, go down—and that's what really matters.

A Single Plate Really Means Less

In the book *Mindless Eating*, Dr. Brian Wansink describes a study he conducted at the Cornell Food and Brand Lab.[1] Two groups of participants were given a meal. One group was told to go into the kitchen and preplate their food; they could put as much as they wanted on their plates, but could do so only once. The other group was allowed to refill their plates as often as they liked. Predictably, the preplaters served themselves much bigger initial portions than the refillers. But when Wansink's team measured how much food each group had consumed at the end of the meal, the refillers had gone back for enough seconds and thirds to consume 14 percent more total calories.

I don't know if it's fair to extrapolate from this one experiment to society at large, but 14 percent more calories is almost enough to account for the obesity epidemic in and of itself (according to the U.S. Department of Agriculture, average daily calorie consumption has risen by 16 percent since 1976).[2] This simple, moderate change in behavior has the potential to make a big difference.

The Power of an Empty Plate

An empty plate sends a powerful, Pavlovian signal to the brain. As you build the habit of limiting yourself to just one, an empty plate will mean "done" on a deep, unconscious level. It's like a stop sign, not only to your conscious brain but also to your appetite. You won't just *know* you're done, you'll *feel* it. "1 = done": very simple, very natural, very powerful.

The sight of an empty plate actually makes you feel full. Appetite responds to visual cues to a far greater degree than most of us imagine. Some other diets encourage people to leave food on their plates at the end of a meal in an effort to break this connection, but why not work *with* this powerful preexisting association rather than against it?

In *Mindless Eating*, Wansink describes another experiment in which he fed each of his research subjects a single bowl of soup—except that some of these bowls weren't really single: they had a secretly attached hose that constantly refilled them. They were, in effect, bottomless soup bowls; they stayed full no matter how much the subjects in front of them ate. And so they kept eating and eating (a whopping 73 percent more than the controls without hoses) simply because they didn't get the visual cue of an empty bowl to tell them to stop.

Does Plate Size Matter?

Don't worry about overloaded plates. Yes, it is possible to put a lot of food onto one plate, but it isn't possible to do so without seeing that it's a lot. The sight of that excess is embarrassing, even just to yourself. When it's all right there in front of you, on one plate, you can't deceive yourself into thinking that you aren't eating a lot. By forcing that excess into the open, you'll gradually shame yourself into smaller portions. Shame tends to get a bad rap these days. It's one of those old-fashioned negative moral terms that is supposed to be the enemy of that modern *summum bonum*, a good self-image. But shame is powerful, it's deep, it's part of human nature, it isn't going away. So you might as well use shame instead of pretending it isn't there. Make it your ally, and maybe shame will even help you deserve a good self-image.

I feel like the Gordon Gekko of self-help writing this, but *shame is good*—or at least, it can be, if you let it. If you don't, it'll still come, uninvited, and then it won't be good at all.

If you are snacking all day long, shame in this positive sense doesn't work. You sneak around any observation, even your own. The irony is you wind up feeling plenty of shame, of course: not at your behavior (which deserves it) but at its results.

That being said, once you have some practice, I think you will be surprised at how well you can eyeball the right amount of food. There will be some big meals the first week or so, but it'll be obvious that they are big. And the slight, mostly unconscious pressure of this obviousness will be enough to gradually whittle them down to size.

Overloaded plates are actually a positive help when you are starting out. They will ensure that you are full enough to make it through to the next meal without snacking. This is important, because getting the "mealing" habits down is more important than caloric restriction up front. The habits are machines that automatically keep churning away, restricting your food consumption long after your conscious mind will have tired of paying attention. So if it costs a few extra calories up front in the form of overloaded single plates to build such a machine, think of them as a sound capital investment.

Gradually, you'll get very good at estimating how much food it will take you to make it through to the next meal. Shame will whittle away at your portions if they're too large, and hunger will keep you from making them too small. This is a very valuable skill, and not something any book or manual can teach you. You have to learn it through experience, and the no seconds rule provides a safe, simple structure for acquiring it.

Plates come in various sizes. Some will end up holding more food than others. But calorically speaking, a single meal doesn't matter (habitually speaking, it does, which is why it's so important to be literally strict). Over the course of months, hundreds of single-plate meals will add up to a substantially smaller amount of food than the same number of multiple-plate meals, and that's really all you ought to care about.

People might point to phenomena such as supersizing as evidence that visual portion control doesn't work, but I disagree. For one thing, supersizing wouldn't be possible without creative packaging. I challenge you to find a plate that would accommodate a supersize McDonald's meal without some serious vertical stacking. (And yes, that means anything that restaurant owners have the gall to *call* a supersize counts as an S; how convenient that it even starts with the letter S!) But, more important, supersizing is evidence of the psychological stopping power of a single plate—if it weren't so powerful, you'd just go ahead and order two bags of fries instead of having to sneak both into one double serving. The fast-food industry is not dumb. They put a lot of research and money into figuring out what it takes to make you eat (and spend) more. Learn from this research and use these insights to do the opposite.

A Normal-Looking Plate

The definition of *normal* is a little like Supreme Court Justice Potter Stewart's definition of pornography: "I know it when I see it." Literally. Because you are limited to single plates, you can actually do effective eyeballing of quantity, which you don't have a prayer at if you're snacking all day long. So, yes, it's possible to stack enormous quantities onto a single plate, but it will be very obvious to you that you are eating a lot of food. If you are determined to sabotage yourself, you could continue to do this; but I think most of us would be a little embarrassed and would try to reduce the vertical dimension a bit.

Not specific enough? How about this: If you have more than one vertical layer of food on your plate, you are almost certainly overeating. So if the bread fits on your plate without covering something else up, you're golden. Is it a disaster to pile on once in a while if the alternative is breaking the *no seconds/no snacks* rule? No. Should you do it regularly? No, you shouldn't. Will you, despite your better knowledge? I don't think so, unless you live by yourself in a cave. Because even if your eyeballing skills are nonexistent, other people will let you know ("Hungry, today, huh?"). Spouses are particularly helpful in this regard. When I started out I piled on some enormous firsts and, because of the looks I got, had to explain (somewhat absurdly) that this was part of my diet. But ah, the power of shame. How nice to have it working for you for a change! I very rarely find myself having to make such explanations anymore.

What If I'm Still Hungry?

If you're still hungry after eating your plateful, then learn from the experience and put more on your plate next time. Learning to eyeball how much is enough is a very important skill, and there's no way to learn it except by being a little hungry a few times. And don't worry: Hunger is a very effective teacher. You'll learn fast. Besides the right amount of food, you'll also learn which kinds of foods fill you up best.

That might be small comfort if you're salivating now as you read this, so try to imagine that the hunger you're feeling is the awareness of calories being burned and that this uncomfortable sensation is a symptom of a very good thing.

Not convinced? Well, you've got a point. Though it can be a motivating fiction to imagine we can feel calories being burned, the truth is that we can't. So try some enlightened self-mockery to put your pangs in perspective. A little temporary hunger between meals isn't going to kill you. And the hunger you're experiencing is really very little by historical standards. People who really go hungry throughout the world wouldn't even recognize what you're feeling as hunger; that's how they probably felt after the best meal of their lives.

Your hunger feels irresistible to you only because you have very little power of resistance. It's only because you're so weak that this feather of hunger is enough to knock you down; in itself, it's not a strong force at all. Here's where the "enlightened" part comes in. I'm not pointing this out to get you down about how weak you are but to show you how weak your opponent is: If you could just get yourself a little bit stronger, you could send him shuffling off with a glance. And nothing builds power like practice. When you resist these pangs, it isn't just a one-time act of virtue, it builds the muscle of resistance. After a few such workouts, next time this wimpy bully hunger comes along to kick sand in your face, he's going to be in for quite a surprise.

When you resist your appetite once, you make future resistance easier. You establish a precedent for good behavior that paves the way for more. It's hard to stay motivated when a bag of chips is just a bag of chips. The stakes seem so small, the gratification so near. But when you look at your decision like this—as precedent—the stakes are higher; the bag of chips represents, to a degree, all future bags of chips. Your resistance now really means something.

Are all these considerations still not enough to motivate you to hold out? Then it's time to move beyond mere pep talk and resort to physical interventions. Have a noncaloric drink. Or even a caloric drink (as long as it isn't sugar soda); protein-rich milk is especially effective in this regard. Whatever it takes to keep to the literal rules and see you through to the next meal without snacking on solid food.

Can I Really Fill Up
My Plate with Anything?

You can put anything—healthy or unhealthy, caloric or not—on your plate, as long as it's not a sweet. Yes, you'll occasionally have an overloaded or unhealthy plate. But we're not worried about being penny-wise here. We're worried about the big picture, about building your habit. And the obviousness of unhealthy, supercaloric, and overflowing plates will act as a very effective disincentive; not every time, but often enough. All you have to worry about is sticking to the one-plate rule and let the rest take care of itself.

Virtual Plates

Sometimes, mostly for social reasons, it isn't possible to fit your entire meal on a single physical plate. Maybe you're at a buffet that has tiny, appetizer-size plates; maybe you're at some kind of banquet where multiple courses are being served; maybe you're at a restaurant where they bring out a separate salad before the entree; maybe you've been invited over to dinner at a friend's house and you don't want to be a demanding guest. For these situations, there's an advanced No S Diet maneuver called "virtual plating" that makes it possible to retain some of the moderating power and integrity of the no seconds rule without offending anyone or making a scene.

It works like this: Instead of relying on a physical plate, you *imagine* a regular-size plate and use that as your limit. As long as what you're eating *could* fit on your imaginary plate, you're okay. If possible, I would suggest making this as concrete as possible by clearing out an area of your physical plate to make room to visually accommodate your next fractional portion.

Virtual plating is an advanced maneuver, and I would recommend saving it for unusual situations like buffets and parties. If it's a celebration, it might be preferable simply to call it an S day (a special day) or even just to chalk it up as a one-time-only failure. You don't want to run the risk of normalizing virtual plating. It's a way to technically bend the rules when you'd otherwise have to break them and it's still not ideal. There is a lot of potential for self-deception and abuse, and habit is never going to understand something this complicated.

Does Fruit Have to Fit on My Plate?

Fruit should fit on your plate. I eat fruit as part of my single-plate meals, and I eat plenty of it. Bulky, healthy fruit is good not only in itself but also because of the real estate it takes up on your plate, displacing less healthy stuff. If you ate fruit between meals, you'd be tempted to skip the fruit at mealtime and put something much less nutritious there instead.

You can also virtually plate your fruit. In other words, if you're going to have a piece of fruit right before or after the rest of your meal, and you think it's barbaric to place an orange next to your filet mignon, leave a conspicuous place for the orange on your plate, an empty spot where it could have fit. That way you're not using the fruit to justify some excessive and/or unhealthy part of your meal.

But as always, virtual plating should be used with

caution. It's usually better to be a little uncivilized and put the orange next to your steak than to risk compromising your new habits.

What About Bread?

Bread (and dinner rolls) should fit on your plate. I'm not a low-carbist, but bread does have calories and plenty of them; it doesn't deserve any special exemptions. If it's part of your meal, it should fit right there on your plate with everything else.

What About Salad?

Salad can go on your main plate. Really, try to do this; it keeps things simpler. If you must eat salad on a separate plate, leave a corresponding void in your main plate, as described above in the "Virtual Plates" section.

What About Soup?

Soup can confound the clarity of No S a bit; it's certainly a mainstream, normal, and acceptable component of the everyday meal and is not something it would be fair to restrict to S days. And yet it often involves an extra plate.

But with a modicum of attention you can pull it off without much trouble. Here's how: (1) If the soup is hearty, have a hunk of bread with it and call it a meal. (2) Or use a smaller dinner plate to compensate for the soup if it is only part of the meal (this is a form of virtual plating). I've done both, but I usually do the first. I eat plenty of soup.

What About Restaurants and Supersizes?

Restaurants raise some problems when it comes to the no seconds rule. Many restaurants now serve plates of food that are really platters—big enough to feed a whole family. Their business is to sell you more food, after all; and if you're not going to ask twice, they'll just give you twice as much the first time you ask. Very smart, from a business perspective. Very dumb, from a diet perspective.

You can bemoan this situation and curse the restaurant industry till you're blue in the face, but these are the facts on the ground. If you want to get and stay thin, you're going to have to deal with them as they are. And don't take it personally. They don't *want* us to get fat, after all, they just want to make money. To them, the obesity epidemic is just a regrettable side effect (and, in fact, for them it's incredibly bad PR).

Ray Kroc, the über-entrepreneur who built up McDonald's from a local mom-and-pop burger joint to the symbol of global capitalism, was *surprised* that people who wouldn't ask for two orders of fries would happily buy one order that was twice as big. He had to be convinced by marketing studies that human beings are really that pathetically self-deceptive. He wasn't some satanic figure bent on seeing the worst in people; but, being a good businessman, he let himself be convinced by overwhelming evidence.

The truth is, there is nothing mysterious or surprising or deceptive about the fact that scarfing down double cheeseburgers and monster orders of french fries will make us fat. If there is any deception going on, it's our own self-deception. Restaurants just need to provide a bit of cover—two portions rolled into one—and we'll hide behind it of our own free will.

On one level, the supersize phenomenon shows how powerful the one-plate rule is: Restaurant owners realized that people are inherently embarrassed to order multiple plates, so they sought to work around this inhibition. With the No S Diet, you use this inhibition as a positive force rather than subverting it. If it's good enough to make McDonald's billions and billions, it's good enough to lose you a few pounds.

Still, it can be tricky when our own strategy is being used against us. So how should a No S Dieter handle eating in restaurants where the plates are as big as platters?

1. The obvious answer is not to eat at these restaurants quite so often. If you eat a platter-size plate once in a blue moon, who cares? You don't need to come up with an explicit, rule-based solution, because it's insignificant. That's more or less how I handle it, but I understand that won't work for everyone.

2. Luckily, not all restaurants serve such big plates, and those that do usually have some smaller dishes as well. So the second option is to do some reconnaissance and find out which plates at which establishments are still reasonably sized. If you eat a few big plates in the process, that's okay, as long as you learn from the experience and avoid them in the future.

3. If you find yourself sitting in front of a gigantic plate and want to redeem the situation, don't be shy about asking for a doggy bag. Weird as it may seem at first if you're not the kind of person who normally does this, you'll feel like a hero when you're walking out the door (if you want an appreciative audience for your heroic act of moderation, post about it to the Nosdiet.com bulletin board).

4. Obviously, avoid anything explicitly labeled as supersize (or whatever euphemism they come up with for it next). That that's an S goes without saying. Try fitting a supersize meal on a plate sometime. Even though there's not a vegetable in sight, it's a challenge. The packaging makes it look deceptively small. A supersize is seconds rolled into firsts.

As more and more people eat this way, insisting on normal-size plates and portions, restaurant owners will respond; they'll have to, if they want to stay in business. (In fact, as I write this, the restaurant chain TGI Fridays is launching a smaller serving size campaign called the "right size.") The No S Diet works well even in the suboptimal social conditions we find now, but my hope is that as more people learn to eat moderately again, those social conditions will change and make it even easier. This isn't a crazy hope; remember, social conditions used to be this way, more or less, all over the place and not so long ago.

5

Days That Start with S

Safety Valve, Reward, Incentive

Most people, no matter what their diet plan is, make exceptions to it from time to time. Holidays, social obligations, or the simple, overwhelming desire to free oneself from eating restrictions eventually break down the most rigorous intentions. Because these exceptions aren't planned, they feel like failures, and dieters get confused and discouraged. On other occasions, when dieters successfully resist the temptation to make an exception, they feel resentful, as if the diet were preventing them from enjoying life. It's a constant struggle between guilt and resentment, with guilt (and failure) usually winning in the end.

The No S Diet is different. Not only does it budget for these exceptions but it uses them as a positive force to prove the rules. Regular breaks are built into the system, not as a necessary evil to be tolerated but as a positive requirement.

How can something negative—not following the rules—be a positive help? In a nutshell: It's a safety valve to keep you from feeling too constrained, a reward for having complied with the rules during the week, and an incentive for you to keep on complying. In fact, I'd go so far as to say that the exception is the most important part of the No S Diet.

Here's how it works: On days that start with the letter S (Saturdays, Sundays, and special days [defined later in this chapter]), you are exempt from the rules, and you can eat whatever you want. This is very simple but very powerful and in ways that may not be immediately obvious. Let me explain.

First off, the terms of the exception are very clear. Just look at the calendar, and you'll know when you can take it and when you can't. This clarity is powerful. It means you'll have a hard time abusing or extending the exception without it being very obvious what you are doing. It limits the scope for self-deception. Yes, you can abuse this rule by counting your hamster's second cousin's birthday as an S day or by gorging yourself with gallons of ice cream every weekend, but you can't do it without knowing you're being a bozo. And most of us, most of the time, will not *knowingly* be bozos.

In most people's minds, dieting equals deprivation.

It's a kind of necessary misery. Either you make yourself miserable by cutting out pleasures entirely or you make yourself miserable by painstakingly counting them and rationing them out in pitiful little doses. Not so with the No S Diet, not with this exception.

Because you know that no food is completely prohibited, just delayed, you don't feel stifled. You don't look at the bowl of ice cream your coworker is eating during the week and think, "My God, I'm never going to be able to eat that again," building up more and more desire and resentment until you break down and gorge on a tub of Ben & Jerry's in a fit of anger and self-pity. You know that all you have to do is wait until the weekend. That knowledge makes it much easier to resist temptation; in fact, that knowledge turns the temptation into an incentive. Your coworker's ice cream isn't a stumbling block to trip you up anymore; instead, it's a symbol of what you have to look forward to. You can have something even *better*. You've got a whole week to plan and prepare. And even if you wind up eating the exact same thing you saw your coworker eating, you'll enjoy it more because of the built-up anticipation of having looked forward to it during the week, and—because instead of furtively scarfing it down as you might have done otherwise—you can enjoy it with a clear conscience, without guilt, as something deserved, even earned. So even on a purely hedonistic level, the No S Diet works: You will enjoy your food more. And if you're a fat person, presumably that is a material consideration. It certainly was for me.

The No S Diet takes the weakness of a sweet tooth

and turns it into a positive, motivating force. The thing that would have made you miserable with longing as an absolute prohibition becomes an incentive when it's merely delayed, dangling in front of you to lead you on to more good behavior. Not only won't you feel deprived but you'll have another reason to succeed. It takes that natural human desire for occasional excess, a desire that normally gets lumped in together with vice, and turns it into a prop for virtue. It makes pleasure good again—usefully good.

Which brings me to another point: Pleasure is good, in itself, not just as a means to something else. And it's an important good, one that's sadly neglected and misunderstood today. On the one hand, puritanical dieters jettison pleasure without a second thought; they'd probably jettison pleasure even if they didn't think it were necessary, just out of a sense of obligatory masochism. On the other hand, high-living hedonists pay lip service to pleasure, but you get the sense that it's really the feeling of badness, of excess, that they relish more than anything else, and that a legitimate pleasure wouldn't even register on their burned-out, jaded taste buds.

But legitimate, moderate pleasure beats the spicy trash of excess hands down—even considered just as pleasure. Instead of always having to top the last excess, you can enjoy every meal in itself. You become awake to the joys of the ordinary and start to wonder whether those extraordinary joys were really joys at all.

The S day exception has a kind of inherent equilibrium. No matter how much you indulge on the weekend, come Monday the slate is clean again. There is no guilt or obligation hanging over you to drag down your morale. Accounting diets sort of let you make exceptions by permitting very sweet and rich foods as long as you balance the books by extreme restriction at some point, but it's easy to make so many exceptions that there's no way you're ever going to be able to balance the books again, creating a caloric bankruptcy, a personal Enron. With the No S Diet, there is no scope for creative accounting or "cooking the books," because there are no books. There is no keeping track of anything besides the day of the week.

The divide between normal days (N days) and S days is a very natural one, and it jibes well with the way society is set up. Most of us work during the week and not on weekends and holidays. It's a powerful, preexisting, externally supported rhythm that the No S Diet and other good habits can tap into. The No S Diet asks only that you think of rules and routine when you are already in that frame of mind, when you're also engaged in the rules and routines of working life, and it lets you relax when you are already relaxing. It demands that you comply only when you're best prepared to comply and doesn't make any demands of you when it would be most difficult, a very efficient use of your limited reserves of willpower.

✱ There is no keeping track of anything besides the day of the week.

What Qualifies as an S Day?

Saturday, Sunday, and special days = S days. Special days include (your) national and (your) religious holidays, and the birthdays of (your) close family and friends. My apologies to atheists and non-native English speakers. A lean and hungry look becomes you. (Just kidding; Sunday is still an S day even if you call it, say, *Domingo*.)

Sick days also start with S. Though I don't imagine you'll be too hungry if you're really sick, you officially have license to do whatever it takes to get better.

Reminder: Throughout this book (and especially in this chapter) I refer to NON-S days (or "normal" days) as N days.

Can I Really Eat Anything on S Days?

You can eat whatever you want on S days. There is no limit. You are free to eat whatever and however much you want—snacks, sweets, seconds, the works. But because of the good habits you've established on weekdays, you'll soon find that you want a lot less.

I understand that this might sound a little scary—being alone with your appetite for days at a time without any rules to prop you up. But it's also quite liberating. It's like riding a bike without training wheels. Sure, you'll fall down a few times at first, but you will learn to ride. And then you'll feel like an adult, a free human being. Even if it's only for a short time, two days a week, you deserve that feeling. Don't deprive yourself of it altogether. At least give it a try. Don't simply assume that you can't do it or jump to conclusions from one or two excessive episodes.

Look, I suppose it is theoretically possible to undo all your good behavior during the week by excessive eating on weekends, but it's not something that could happen by accident, without your noticing. Because of your training during the week, every time you reach for snacks, sweets, or seconds, you'll be very conscious of what you're doing. It will seem strange. That sense of strangeness, along with a genuinely diminished appetite from having become accustomed to eating less, and just a *touch* of common sense, will usually be enough to get you through your S days without undue excess. My S days tend to be no worse than my ordinary days were before I started the No S Diet.

How Do I Avoid Binging on S Days?

Binging on S days is less of an issue than you might think. I haven't heard of anyone messing this diet up because they followed the rules during the week and binged on the weekends. But I have heard from plenty of people who anticipate this being a problem, burden themselves with weekend restrictions to prevent it, and then crack during the week because it's too much. S days are a necessary reward and safety valve.

As one successful No S Dieter succinctly put it: "S days should be S days so that N days aren't."

Binging is a psychological reaction against deprivation. But on the No S Diet you aren't really depriving yourself of anything worth mentioning during the week, you're eating three solid meals a day. So your binge instinct doesn't really have anything to react against. N days are about *moderation*, not deprivation. A pendulum that stops sort of in the middle isn't going to swing back very far in the opposite direction, if at all. It may take you a few weekends to really get this; but when you do, your binging days are over.

Still, people starting out on the No S Diet tend to worry about undoing all their good moderate behavior during the week with immoderate eating on weekends and holidays. I don't think this is actually much of an issue long term—both because of the psychological reasons I just discussed and because weekday habits soon start carrying over to S days. But if people get discouraged by short-term S day excess and quit, well then they'll never get to the long term. So here are some tricks for keeping S days relatively moderate without burdening yourself with additional restrictions (which would really make you want to binge).

Reward Away Resentment

If you want to be proactive, ward off binges by actively rewarding yourself with the treat you want most instead of hunkering down and hoping you don't get too hungry. If your appetite feels properly taken care of, it's less likely to revolt. You'll enjoy yourself more, and your appetite will appreciate the gesture of respect. It will cease simmering and plotting revenge at the first opportunity. Remember, binging is mostly about revenge—don't give your appetite the pretext for it. Proactively rewarding yourself is win–win; you'll wind up eating less and enjoying it more. It's counterintuitive but very effective (and pleasurable).

Don't Stress About S Day Overeating

Overeating is going to happen on some weekends, especially at the beginning, when your body hasn't become habituated to eating less. Don't let this upset you too much. As your weekday habits improve, they'll unconsciously carry over to the weekend. Snacking will no longer be automatic; you'll be full sooner because you've been eating less; and sweets will taste sweeter so you require less to get your fix. You'll still probably eat more on the weekends, but it will be less more than before. Sort of miraculously obvious, isn't it?

Keep the Focus on N Days

The best way to compensate for an excessive weekend is not to add extra rules but to redouble your vigilance about adhering to the existing rules during the week. This is important not only in the direct sense that there are far more weekdays than weekends and holidays, but also indirectly because your actions on N days will start to unconsciously affect your behavior on S days.

So don't be discouraged if you have a really excessive S day now and then. It will happen, especially at the beginning. Discouragement is the real danger. As long as you follow the N day rules over the long term, the extra calories of an occasional excessive S day won't matter.

Is It Extra-Good
to Take Fewer S Days?

It's extra-*bad* to skip S days. This is another example of the perfect being the enemy of the good. You need

S days. Even just as concession to your appetite; they're a necessary concession because your appetite will take revenge without them. But they're more than that, too. They are a pleasure, a real, legitimate, powerful pleasure, and that's worth something. This pleasure is what will allow you to stay on the No S Diet over the long haul. If you didn't have that safety valve, the steam would build up and you'd break down into unscheduled, unenjoyed, self-loathing binges and eventually give up on the diet altogether.

It's easy to misdiagnose excessive S days as a problem. What you do on N days is much, much more important, and the (relatively) free and enjoyable S days are critical to that. You have only so much willpower, and it goes a lot farther on N days. Be careful that your S day worries aren't an excuse to overextend yourself and fail.

So take the full complement of *legitimate* S days— weekends, national and religious holidays, special birthdays—and enjoy them without reservation. You can't be virtuous without this pleasure. It's your duty. Enjoy.

What If I Mess Up During the Week?

If you mess up during the week, you might be tempted to "make up for it" by giving up an S day. But it's a terrible idea to trade days after the fact, as revenge for a failure. That just gives you license to fail again. By paying off a debt, you're mentally opening up a line of credit: You'll always think you can make up for a weekday excess later, so the bar for breaking the rules will be much lower. By making failure correctable you also make it much more likely. It's hard enough to resist that brownie without hearing a little devil whisper in your ear, "Go ahead, enjoy, you can always make up for it later!"

And if you're having trouble making it through the week, the last thing you want to do is give yourself an extra opportunity for failure on the weekend. In college, if you fail a basic physics course, the solution isn't to take advanced physics, but to take the basic physics course over again until you get it right. It's the same basic principle here, except there's nothing but your better judgment to stop you from doing it. You have no business worrying about S days if you can't even do N days right.

In Chapter 6, I discuss a number of ways to handle failure, and trading days emphatically isn't one of them. Please take a look there before you start, because most of us—all of us, probably—are going to mess up in some way at some point, and how we react to that failure is more important than the failure itself.

Can I Trade Days in Advance?

Officially, there is no trading S days ahead of time, either. Swapping is usually more dangerous than it's worth. Still, I say "not officially" instead of "no" because I understand that there are times when it makes sense. For example, when there are a bunch of legitimate and mandatory non-weekend special days all at once—for example, multiple birthdays and the holiday season. But, in general, if it's a genuinely special day, then take an S day. No need to trade.

One of the powerful things about the N day/S day divide is its clarity. When you start trading days, you muddy this clarity. "S-ing" on an N day will no longer seem taboo.

So when you're confronted with a temptation that you're contemplating trading for, either declare that day an S day, chalk it up as a failure, or resist it. If it obviously doesn't seem S-day worthy, use that knowledge to give you the strength to resist.

What Does a Perfect S Day Look Like?

A perfect S day isn't a day when somehow, without any rules, you managed not to eat any snacks, seconds, or sweets. You don't have to be a saint. Nor is it a day when you gorged yourself on every imaginable restricted delicacy that you couldn't enjoy during the week, taking full advantage of the lack of rules like a looter during a blackout.

A perfect S day is when you've basically stuck with your weekday three-meal rhythm but have added an extra reward, something especially nice, and enjoyed it without reservation or guilt. As I've said, these two things are related: Counterintuitive as it may seem, the reward promotes the moderation.

✱ The reward promotes the moderation.

Can I Fail on an S Day?

There is no such thing as a failed S day, even if you do wind up wolfing down an unconscionable amount of food. So do not stress if you have an S day—especially in the beginning—that does not in any way, shape, or form resemble the perfect S day I just described. *The habits that you build during the week will start to carry over to the weekend*, as long as you're patient and stick with it.

If your S days are more about quantity than quality, plan ahead. Make sure you *don't* have so much quantity around and that you *do* have some quality. Be proactive about quality. Don't skimp. Give yourself the best, what you most want. And don't wait. Do it before you're eating the carpet.

The quality will take the edge off your hunger, and remove any resentment. It will also leave your wallet a little emptier, which is helpful if, like me, you can't afford *both* quality and quantity.

What If I Work Weekends?

If your days off from work are not on the weekends, you might be wondering whether it makes sense to permanently switch and make them your exempt S days instead, even though they don't start with the letter S. I hate to disappoint you, but the answer is "it depends."

Switching your fixed S days is more dangerous than keeping them Saturday and Sunday because you'll be tempted to take weekend S days, too (especially if you do most of your socializing then). But, realistically, if that's your work schedule, it might be your best option. There are pros and cons either way. You have to decide what's personally more important to you: enjoying your days off to the max or not having to resist the sibilant social siren song of days that actually start with S.

What About Vacation?

Vacation isn't much of an issue for American wage slaves like myself; there just isn't a whole lot of damage you can do in a mere two weeks. Citizens of more enlightened countries may want to consider it more closely.

Here's one way to go about it: If you're lucky enough to be enjoying a long vacation, try to make each weekday vacation day an N day, but if you know in advance that there's something really special and worth making an exception for (say you're in Italy and are anticipating some local delicacy), declare it an S day and enjoy.

How Many Non-Weekend S Days Can I Take?

There's no hard limit to the number of special days you can take because people from different countries with different religions and different social circles celebrate different holidays. Sometimes these may fall all at once within a narrow time frame. But I'd say if you're consistently taking more than two non-weekend special days a month, you may want to consider clamping down a bit.

Don't obsess about keeping track of non-weekend S days, and don't worry at all about this if your N day behaviors are good and you're happy with the results you're seeing. However, if you've been on the No S Diet for a while and your N day behaviors have been perfect, but the scale isn't responding, you *might* want to look at the number of non-weekend S days you are taking. I hesitate to recommend this; I do it mostly just to preempt the question, because most of the people who worry about S days can't even manage to behave properly on N days and should really stay focused on that. This is an advanced worry. Make sure you have the basics down first.

Season's Warnings

Thanksgiving, Christmas, New Year's—"the Holidays." It's a wonderful time of year, but not for dieting.

Why is that? It's only a few days. If you count Christmas Eve as a legitimately excessive day, it's just five days in four months, counting from Halloween: Halloween, Thanksgiving, Christmas Eve, Christmas Day, and New Year's Eve. It shouldn't make that much of a difference. (If you're Jewish, you might want to limit Hanukkah S days to one or two crazy nights.)

Of course, it *isn't* just five excessive days for most people. If it were, there wouldn't be a problem. But because of all the leftovers, people continue eating at celebratory levels many days after Thanksgiving and Halloween. Then they go to a gazillion holiday parties and overeat there, too. And even when they aren't staring at leftovers or bowls of eggnog, they think, "I've overeaten so much already, why restrain myself now? I might as well cram it all in until it's time to get virtuous again for my New Year's resolution."

I actually think it is the latter part of that, thinking, "Why bother? I might as well wait till New Year's to fix it" that is the bigger problem. The leftovers and Christmas parties are a bit of a problem in themselves, but they're mostly just an excuse for this flopping out altogether. They're pretexts for outraged perfectionism and laziness to seize on. Still, they are problems, even if largely as excuses, so we have to deal with them.

The way to deal with leftovers and holiday parties is very simple: clarity. This is where the N day/S day structure is particularly useful.

Decide what your S days are up front, and stick with them. Write them down, if you think it will help. Mark them in your calendar. Just the fact that you've made a clear, firm, reasonable decision is enormously powerful. It's not going to solve the problem for you, but it's a lever that makes it possible for your puny daily will-power to succeed.

In terms of clarity, leftovers are easy. If you're doing the No S Diet, you clearly can eat them *only* as part of a single-plate meal and *only* if they're not sweets. If this clarity isn't enough, get rid of them. Better the trash can at the curb than the trash can of your stomach.

Throwing out food is hard for some people, I understand this. I don't like it either. If the trash can is too harsh, give it away. Bring it to work and inflict it on

---

✳ Decide what your S days are up front, and stick with them.

your coworkers. Freeze it. Put it in a basket and float it down the River Nile.

You either have to learn to resist leftovers or to get over your squeamishness and get rid of them. If you don't want to be fat, you have no alternative.

It's the social events that can get really tricky. There will probably be at least a couple more days besides the big five S days that you'll more or less have to take as special days: a holiday family get-together or an office holiday party, for instance. And that's okay in itself. A day or two more isn't going to kill you. The danger is the damage that those extra days can do to your clearly defined boundaries. So take the days; you really don't have a choice. But keep your eye on the boundaries. It's tricky, but you can deal with this issue if you're careful.

One method is to count the extra S days; if you have more than two, slam on the brakes and accept that there might be a little social awkwardness at your next get-together. Generally speaking, I'm against counting stuff; but if you think you're likely to be derailed by excessive holiday S days, the payout in terms of self-discipline might be worth it. You might even want to go further and use a calendar and colored markers to mark off each day as a success (in green), a failure (in red), or an exempt S day (in yellow), a technique I'll describe in Chapter 6. Keeping such a "habit calendar" makes sense any time of year, but it is particularly useful and appropriate—think Advent calendar—during the holidays.

Okay, so much for the excuses. Now for the harder part: how to avoid giving up entirely until January 1 if you run into trouble. You might have a day or two when you've just screwed up, and your morale is in the toilet. You'll think, "I messed up my winning streak. My sense of perfectionism is outraged. Why not just throw in the towel and wait till New Year's, when Father Time will come around to wipe the slate clean?" You know all the merely rational arguments against this kind of thinking already. But when you've fallen off the wagon, reason and enlightened self-interest often aren't enough, so here are some tricks for salvaging a less than perfect holiday season.

Adjust Your Expectations

Do not expect to lose any weight during this period of time. Your goal should be maintenance. This is reasonable given the temptations and the weather, which is not conducive to calorie-burning activities. Given that most people gain weight over the holidays, just by standing still you are zipping past the Joneses. Most important, this will help prevent disappointment. A minor setback will be much less likely to turn into a rout. And if you do actually lose some weight, you'll be that much more thrilled.

Focus on a Minimum Level of Daily Compliance

Your goal should be making it through each day without breaking the literal rules. Don't worry if some of those firsts were a little large. Don't worry if you really went overboard on a legitimate S day. And above all, don't worry about the scale. Marking off your daily compliance on a habit calendar can be an excellent, concrete method of keeping your focus in the right place.

Wrap Up Goodies for S Days

If you're at a holiday party that doesn't fall on a legitimate S day, keep in mind that you can always wrap up some goodies to take home with you and enjoy on the next S day. This is a great way to get people off your back if they're pressing you to try (say) their special holiday brownies. See page 139 for more advice on how to deal with social pressure in general.

Stop Making New Year's Resolutions

New Year's resolutions are a terrible idea. For one thing, they almost never work, because it's very hard to make plans for such a long time frame. But the worst part, worse than the mere inefficacy of these resolutions, is how they serve as an excuse for putting off necessary self-improvement projects. Get rid of New Year's resolutions, and you can't say to yourself, "I'll just wait till then"; you have to fix the problem now. When you fail, you have to get right back up. There's no time out or waiting period for your perfectionist tabula rasa to get reset.

Don't get me wrong—resolutions are a great thing. A year is just the wrong scale at which to make them. In the next chapter, I'll talk about a much better structure for acquiring good habits (like the No S Diet): making *monthly* resolutions.

6

Building the No S Habit

The Power of Habit

Nothing is more powerful than habit. —Ovid

Habit is overcome by habit. —Thomas à Kempis

Habit is either the best of servants or the worst of masters. —Nathaniel Emmons

Overeating is not the result of a rational thought process. We don't do some kind of (faulty) cost–benefit analysis and *decide* that the pleasure of this bag of cookies is worth what it will do to our gut. And we aren't going to *stop* overeating by means of such a rational cost–benefit analysis either, by simply getting the math right. There is no analysis. It's automatic. It's *habit*. We eat the cookies because that's what we did last time, and the time before, and the time before.... At some point there may have been a rational (or at least conscious) decision involved; but if so, it was a long time ago.

Habit is a funny thing. It's basically the way our minds optimize frequently repeated thought processes. Conscious thought is expensive; it's slow; you can consciously think about only one thing at a time. The mind is parsimonious with conscious thought. It wants to economize, to save conscious thought for novel situations that really require it. So if you make the same decision a few times your mind starts to build a habitual shortcut to bypass some of that premium-level thought next time. It saves the result of the decision in a version of what computer scientists call a "lookup table": For this stimulus, return that response; you don't even have to think about it. Why waste precious conscious thought reworking out a decision that's already been made? Just look up what you did last time. The more you repeat an action, the more conscious thought your mind sees it can save, and the more efficient and automatic the looking up becomes. When you have good responses stored in this table, habit is fantastic; you do the right thing automatically. When you have the wrong responses stored, it's a disaster.

So how do you correct a bad habit like overeating? The first step is by recognizing that it is a habit: something unconscious, automatic, and acquired; something that, although very powerful, can be retrained and made to work for you. Once you've understood this, the next step is obvious: Rewire the association—turn the bad habit into a good one. Precisely how you do this rewiring can be a little tricky, but most commercial diets don't even try: They either ignore the power of habit by confronting your problem of overeating on a purely conscious level, or they have you trick and appease your existing bad habits instead of fundamentally altering them. Neither strategy works.

Taming Habit

A good analogy for understanding how to correct a bad habit is to think of it as wild animal, powerful but dumb. Your rational self is like an animal trainer locked in a cage with a fearsome beast. When you think of habit this way, it also becomes very clear why popular approaches to diet fail.

On forbidden-foods diets, you're told to sneak around your bad habit of overeating by redirecting it toward certain approved foods on which you can continue to gorge. That's like trying to distract a tiger from what he really wants to eat by throwing him scraps of something else. It may work for a while, but eventually the tiger is going to eat what he wants—he's still a wild animal, after all.

On accounting diets, your rational self is asked to

✳ Think of habit as a wild animal, powerful but dumb.

do all the work, counting calories or carbs or points. This task would be hard enough even if your existing bad habits left you alone. But they won't. Those wild animals aren't just going to sit patiently in the cage and watch with detached amusement as you flex your puny mental muscles on the fundamentally physical task of reducing their allotment of kibble. They want precisely the opposite of what your rational, counting self wants; and being much stronger, they'll get it.

On both these kinds of diets, the bad habit of overeating remains intact. And in time, that bad habit is going to get you.

So if you can't beat habit by fighting it head-on and if you can't ignore or appease it either, what's left? To tame it. Human beings do tame elephants, after all, and then ride on their backs and compel them to pull 10-ton logs that a dozen strong men couldn't budge. In the same way, with the right techniques, your conscious mind can tame habit. And habit working *for* you is a remarkable thing.

All it takes is a little carrot and stick. In the rest of this chapter I'll show you how the No S Diet provides these and what you can do to apply them most effectively, so that habit will support rather than undermine your weight-loss efforts.

Habit-Friendly Behaviors

Habits are safer than rules; you don't have to watch them. And you don't have to keep them, either. They keep you.

—Frank Crane, Presbyterian minister

The rules of the No S Diet are great, as far as rules go. They are much easier and more pleasant to comply with than the rules of most other diets. But the best thing about them is how readily they become unconscious habits. The rules prescribe *habit-friendly* behaviors.

What makes a behavior habit friendly? I think you can boil it down to three things. Such behaviors are *natural*, *simple*, and *unobtrusive*.

Natural

As I mentioned in Chapter 1, the behaviors prescribed by the No S Diet are similar to "natural," traditional eating patterns. Most people in most places used to eat like this, more or less. Habit is often called second nature. The fact that these behaviors resemble *first* nature means that the associations that you are trying to build have already been primed. Instead of having to be forced in against a lot of resistance, they'll easily fall into place.

Simple

Wild animals can't do math—and neither can habit. If you don't keep the behaviors you are trying to habitu-alize nice and simple, your conscious mind is going to have to stay involved; habit can't take over. You have to dumb down your problems a bit in order to sim-plify them to the point that habit can deal with them. That means accepting the fact that you aren't going to produce the *perfect* response for every situation. That's okay. You don't need perfect. It would take you hours (if not days, years, or lifetimes) of deliberation to come up with just one meal that perfectly balances the competing concerns of nutrition, taste, sociability, and so on. You need a good enough that is also *simple* enough to offload to habit; and that's what the No S Diet gives you.

Unobtrusive

You don't have just one habit. You've got many. And you've got obligations to the outside world as well, such as your job, family, and hobbies. Your eating habits should conflict with these other habits and obligations to the minimum possible degree. Because if there is conflict, then habit has to turn to the conscious mind for resolution. And if that happens often enough, habit starts to unravel. The No S Diet gives you rules that are so unobtrusive that chances are good that no one else will even notice you are following them unless you tell them. You don't need special food that may or may not be available. You don't need to time anything too precisely. You don't need to do any calculations or to keep track of multiple variables. Except for the bad habit of overeating that it corrects, the No S Diet fits around your other existing habits and obligations. It slides right in.

Strictness Makes It Easier

Strictness sounds so old-fashioned. Unpleasant. Like a mean schoolmarm. It also sounds hard. And it can be all of those things. But it can also be a great and necessary help if you're strict about the right things in the right way.

The basic case for strictness is that it builds habit faster. If you are strict, your appetites learn quickly that it's not worth testing the boundaries all the time. Your habits are like children. If you are not strict or if you are inconsistent, they'll constantly be testing, seeing how far they can go, and you'll actually wind up having to use more willpower to resist them. So paradoxically, strictness makes it easier. It's being lenient that's hard.

When you're strict, there is no decision to be made, no wrangling, no "can I? can't I?" You're pre-*dis*approved, so forget it and move on to something else. The prohibition passes from something merely rational to something reflexive. It becomes automatic and easy.

But isn't strictness dreary and depressing? Not if you are *comically* strict. Acknowledge that there is an element of humorous inflexibility in your decision to avoid (say) a midafternoon carrot stick, and smile at it. Big picture it makes sense, but little picture it is a bit silly, and you might as well have a sense of humor about it.

The No S Diet has exceptions built into it already. You don't need to add any more. If you add more exceptions or are lax about applying the rules, you risk pushing moderate into ineffective. If you're strict about the No S Diet, you're not being cruel to yourself. It is inherently tolerant.

The most important time for strictness is at the beginning, when your habit is new. Later, when your habit becomes mature, strictness won't really be much of an issue. The habit will then do what's right automatically. It will have internalized the strictness.

Fence Around the Diet

There's a Jewish expression, "Build a fence around the law," which means don't do anything that might possibly be interpreted as giving even the appearance of violating sacred law. The idea is that sometimes it's hard to know precisely when an important moral or religious line is being crossed, so you should draw another line farther out. That far-out line may be a little arbitrary, but it's very clear, and if you stop things at that level, you can be confident they haven't crossed a more important, but more ambiguous boundary. And because the far-out line is very clear, it's easy to make fast, snap decisions. A scholar might have the luxury of contemplating the deep subtleties of the underlying law, but for ordinary observant Jews in daily life, the clarity outlined by that fence is critical because other-wise, how could they make the hundreds of practical decisions they have to make every day?

I hope no one will consider it blasphemous that I apply this religious principle to profane matters such as weight loss, because I think it's based on a profound and useful psychological insight, and it's with great respect that I repurpose it here.

Here's an example of how the No S Diet makes use of this fence around the law principle: I don't eat snacks, not even healthy ones. Would it really be so bad if I ate a pomegranate before dinner, just this once? Pomegranates are a super-health food, and one would be good for me, probably, in itself. But I don't. Because *nothing is in itself*. If I ate the pomegranate, I'd start having to wonder all the time about whether this food or that food was worth making an exception for. It would smudge the clarity of the rule. Even if I tended to make good choices (which I doubt I would), it would just be too expensive in terms of mental resources. I've got better things to think about. And there's no way I'm going to be able to train unconscious habit to make sophisticated decisions like this.

How strict should you be? The stricter you are, the faster your habits will take hold. I find the fence around the law analogy helpful because it keeps me from trying to evaluate potential exceptions on a case-by-case basis. It keeps me from getting into an internal argument with myself every time I'm confronted with some little-picture "good in itself" potential exception that risks my hard-won habits. They are taboo, not to be reasoned about. Reason is wonderful, but expensive. Save it for more worthwhile pursuits.

Recovering from Failure

Strictness is important. But strictness does not mean punishment. Nor does it mean compensating for failures by being extra-good in the future. It just means being very clear as to what constitutes success and failure, trying your best to meet the criteria for success, and being honest with yourself when you fail to meet them.

Punishment and restitution are actually bad and counterproductive. I don't say this from some kind of mushy "love yourself," "I'm okay, you're okay" perspective. On the contrary, I say it because when you punish yourself or try to make amends for having messed up, what you're really doing, at a deep psychological level, is saying, "It's all right to fail because I can make up for failure later." You think you're just paying off a debt, but you're also, and more importantly, opening up a line of credit. That line of credit, that idea that you can make up for failure in the future, will make you much more likely to fail in the future. You've lowered the stakes; you've lowered the cost of failure; you've lowered the incentive to succeed.

If, on the other hand, you know that you have just one chance to behave correctly, that there is no makeup test, you'll take your behavior much more seriously, and you'll have much better odds of succeeding the first and only time around.

So when you fail, just get up, brush off the dust, pause to consider what you did wrong and how to avoid it going forward, and move on. The positively strict thing to do is *not* to beat yourself up, but to acknowledge that you failed, *without* punishing yourself. Save your strictness for your future self rather than your past. Self-revenge is really a kind of self-indulgence.

Some people get the No S Diet the first time they try it. It works and it sticks. But most people have a bit

✳ Save your strictness for your future self rather than your past.

more trouble than that. In fact, you might do best if you assume you'll screw up the first time, so that you don't get too discouraged. Consider it a reconnaissance mission, a trial run, just to feel out how hard it's going to be and see where problems are going to arise. If the enemy—your appetite—turns out to be such a chump that your reconnaissance mission routs him, great, you've succeeded. It might be that easy; you won't know until you try. If not, you've learned more about this enemy and where he's likely to ambush you. You're stronger and better prepared for next time.

Don't feel stupid for trying and failing. Success is the sum of many failures. This isn't just a pep talk. According to *Washington Post* health columnist Sally Squires:

> *Studies show that altering eating habits for good requires 10 to 12 concerted attempts to succeed— which is to say about a dozen failures come before the eventual success. "That's not reason to despair," said John Norcross, professor of psychology at the University of Scranton in Pennsylvania and a researcher on self-initiated change. "If anything, it's reason to say, 'I'm not doing so bad.'"* [1]

Sometimes it takes a false start (or 12). So quit dawdling and get some failures under your belt!

If that statistic is insufficiently inspiring, I'll close this section on a more eloquent note with a quote from Winston Churchill (not, admittedly, the thinnest man in the world, but he did have some pretty serious problems that he managed to overcome): "Success consists of going from failure to failure without loss of enthusiasm."

Setting Expectations

The great thing about the moderate, sustainable weight loss that you'll experience on the No S Diet is that it is so painless. You aren't really sacrificing anything. In fact, most people find they start to enjoy eating more than ever did before, without obsessing about it. The downside to this comfortable pace is that it is slow. It takes patience to see results. That can be difficult. So it's best to brace for this up front and set your expectations accordingly.

There are two kinds of expectations most of us have about diet: *What* we will see, and *when* we will see it; i.e., time and results. And most of us are looking for the wrong thing on both of these counts.

Regarding time, do not think in terms of days and weeks. Think in terms of months and years. Even better, think in terms of the rest of your life. It probably took you a long time to get fat; it's only to be expected that it's going to take a long time to get you thin again. And the harder, more important part is staying thin once you get there. So start worrying about that problem now. Maintenance is more important than progress. And the more you focus on it up front, the better your long-term prospects.

Maintenance is more important than progress.

Regarding results, do not think in terms of pounds lost on the scale. Sustainable weight loss is about half a pound a week. That's too subtle for you to measure on a daily or even weekly basis on a household scale. You will drive yourself crazy trying and will become demoralized by random fluctuations. Think in terms of behavior instead. If you want to count something to measure progress, count the number of consecutive days you have successfully complied with the No S Diet. I call this metric *Days on Habit*. Better yet, mark off successful N days on a calendar in green, exempt S days in yellow, and failures in red (this is the Habit Traffic Light, discussed later in this chapter).

Put the Scale in Perspective

Some time ago I noticed that a lot of people on the Nosdiet.com bulletin board were becoming obsessed with minor fluctuations in their weight. So I thought I would pay attention to my own weight on the scale for a few days. I was hoping to collect some hard data with which to reassure these people that their fluctuations were not something unusual or bad.

What was the result? I couldn't have made up something better.

The day I started my experiment I weighed 171 pounds. No surprise. On the website I quote my weight as 170. I'm usually a little under when I bother to check, but 171 is about what I'd expect. I stepped on the scale a couple more times to confirm: 171 both times.

The next morning, I stepped on the scale again. This time I was 161 pounds. I had lost 10 pounds in one day. I stepped on the scale a couple more times to confirm. Still 161.

I had done nothing unusual. It was the same time of day, and the same situation, right after breakfast and exercise. And I wasn't even actively trying to lose weight. I've been maintaining a pretty ideal weight for about four years now. And yet, according to my scale, I had lost 10 pounds, overnight, without even trying. It sounds like one of those quick-fix diet ads on the Internet—even better!

Do I believe this number? Do I think it is significant? Or course not. These numbers make no sense. This was obviously just an aberration of the scale, maybe coupled with some digestive issues. But if I had been trying to lose weight, or I had been gorging myself, I might have read these numbers quite differently. Or if I'd just waited a week in between measurements, then those numbers might have seemed to me very meaningful. I might have thought, "Aha, my diet is working!" or "Wow, I can eat like a pig and it doesn't matter!" The numbers would have misled me about my behavior.

So what happened the day after my 10-pound drop? I was back to 170. I'd gained 9 of my 10 pounds back again overnight.

Let me just say that my scale is not particularly awful, from what I can judge from previous experience. It's a reasonably reputable recent-vintage digital scale. It's at least as good as any scale I've previously owned.

You might be thinking, "Well, I have a medical-quality scale that would never be so inaccurate." Maybe you do. Great. That's certainly better. But I've had some bad experiences with medical-quality scales too, scales that were actually in the doctor's office. Our first daughter was a preemie; and right from the beginning, she was off-the-charts small. We made ourselves crazy trying to cram enough calories into her. When she was about six months old, our otherwise wonderful pediatrician told us she was so underweight that we would have to take her to a feeding specialist. In the end, though, it turned out that the problem was with our pediatrician's scale. It was off by more than 10 percent; our daughter was actually fine.

Look, it's nice for me to be able to say, "I've lost 40 pounds" on the No S Diet. I'm not knocking scales completely. But it is absurd and counterproductive for people to prostrate themselves before the scale as if awaiting the infallible judgment of the almighty. I get people posting losses or gains of half a pound on the Nosdiet.com website. There is no way that means anything. Your scale is not that accurate, and even if it were, you might be measuring "time since last bowel movement" rather than anything you really care about. That 10-pound fluctuation I described was unusual. But I have 5-pound fluctuations all the time. And I see lots of people posting jubilantly about 5-pound losses or dejectedly confessing 5-pound gains.

The point I'm trying to make here is not that scales are useless and should never be trusted, but that they are not accurate enough that you should make yourself crazy over day-to-day fluctuations. *Any single measurement is not really worth much.* Scales also don't quite measure the right thing. What we're interested in isn't really weight. It's fat, and fat versus muscle. Weight is just an approximate way of getting at this.

So should you measure waist circumference or something else instead? From what I've read about measuring waist circumference, it does seem like a better metric. But I have to admit, I don't do it. I still step on the scale now and then; that's still the only results-based metric I use. But it's not my primary metric. It's just a rough occasional sanity check, and I do it to make sure the number I quote on the No S Diet website isn't way off. My primary metric is behavioral: *Days on Habit*, as I discuss later in the chapter. And this I think is the primary metric most people should switch to.

How Your Scale Is Like the Stock Market

You might think that the solution to the inaccuracy of any individual scale measurement would be to take a lot of them. But I'm not so sure. Bad news, even if it's small and unreliable, can cause us to react in irrational and disproportionate ways.

In the book *Fooled by Randomness*, Nassim Taleb considers a hypothetical exceptional investor who makes 15 percent a year on average.[2] Sometimes he makes more, sometimes less. In any given year, he's 93 percent likely to have made money. But if you look at any given month, he's only 67 percent likely to have made money. It's even less at the weekly level; and at the daily level, it's only a tad over 50 percent. We're talking about the same overall level of success, just measured at different intervals.

Why is this an important or interesting observation? Because human psychology is such that losses hurt us more than gains give us pleasure. If investors check their investments only once a year, they almost never feel losses. If they check them every day or more, then they feel hundreds of losses. Not only is this unpleasant, but it's likely to drive these investors to make bad, irrational decisions. People tend to feel loss versus gain in binary terms: It's not so much the magnitude of either as the direction. A little loss hurts almost as much as a big one. As a result, most investors would be much better off not checking their stocks at frequent intervals.

What does this have to do with dieting? Consider stepping on a scale. Even if your diet is going very well, if you measure yourself daily, you are going to see some numbers that make you unhappy. Weight doesn't fluctuate like a stock, but it does fluctuate, however virtuously you're adhering to your diet. And if these fluctuations go the wrong way, as they often will, we are hardwired to feel pain. Even if your self-esteem is such that you don't mind being unhappy, consider this: As with stocks, unhappiness isn't conducive to rational decision making. You're that much more likely to overreact, despair of your progress and fall off the wagon. Measuring once a week is better. Once a month is better still. At that time, take the average of several measurements over three days or so—and then stop until next month.

Focus on Behavior, Not Results

When you step on the scale and see a 5-pound gain or loss, what do you do with this information? How do you react? Most people get depressed when they see a bad number—and that all too often leads to emotional

Good behavior comes first.

eating, or binging on comfort food (although *self-hatred* food would be a more accurate description in this case). And when they see a good number, they figure they can relax, take it easy, maybe celebrate a little, and eat a little more. There are people who can take these numbers in stride. But I think these are people who know that the numbers are of secondary importance, that good behavior comes first. What you really see when you step on the scale—distorted by a lot of random noise—is the result of your behavior, good or bad. So why not focus on that directly? The cause instead of the effects.

When you focus on behavior, you get results thrown into the bargain because behavior causes results. When you focus on results, you get neither because results cannot exist without behavior. And behavior, besides being a *better* thing to measure, is also an *easier* thing to measure.

Tracking Progress with the Habit Traffic Light

So it's better to keep track of behavior than results. But how precisely should you do this? With something I call the *Habit Traffic Light*. Here's how it works: The No S Diet gives you three simple rules for how to behave. Every day, you either abide by these rules or you don't; or there's a third possibility, you could be exempt (because it's an S day). So you take a calendar and make a green mark on every day you succeed, a red mark on every day you fail, and a yellow mark for every S day. Green, yellow, red—like a traffic light. It's not a whole lot of effort keep track of this; there's just one data point per day, and at the end of the month you'll have a very striking picture—literally, a picture—of how well you adhered to the behavior you set out to achieve.

Why bother with the Habit Traffic Light? After all, one of the great benefits of the No S Diet is its lack of requirements for keeping track of minutiae. Let's consider what you get for your effort.

The primary benefit of the Habit Traffic Light is motivational. For one thing, seeing the green, yellow, and red marks gives you a feeling of accountability, and that can be powerful. By recording failures, you can't as easily pretend they didn't happen; it's harder to just conveniently forget that you screwed up three days running, and that raises the stakes. More positively, once you have a few green success days under your belt, you don't want to break your winning streak. You feel like you've accumulated something that would be a shame to throw away.

The format makes a difference, too. Coloring in a calendar is visually compelling in a more than rational way. You've heard the saying "A picture is worth a thousand words." That's true motivationally as well. No mere number will inspire you like this image.

A second benefit is diagnostic. Let's say you've done the No S Diet for three months and you haven't lost any weight. You look at the calendar and see a lot of red. Well, it's no mystery why you didn't lose weight. You simply didn't do what you were supposed to do. If, on the other hand, it's solid green (with a bit of S-day yellow) then you can go digging for more profound and subtle explanations (see the next section).

A third benefit is that if you feel the need to keep track of something—and I think a lot of people do—at least keeping track of Days on Habit keeps you focused on behavior, not results. It indulges your "must keep track of something" urge without distracting you from what is directly under your control.

A fourth benefit is that, compared to other scoring systems, the Habit Traffic Light encourages you to consistently strive for a *sustainable minimum of compliance*, rather than heroically overreaching. The best thing you can get with the Habit Traffic Light is success. There's no double success or triple success. And this is important. The goal is regularity, a daily good enough. You don't want some more complex point system that encourages you to balance terrible days with extra-good ones. Because then all you're doing with your extra virtue is buying the license for extra vice. You will get yourself into massive debt that way, wracking up huge vices that you kid yourself into thinking you're going to pay off someday with mighty feats of virtue.

How long should you keep track of your behavior like this? As long as you're worried about it. It takes about 21 days to form a habit, so some people shoot for that. If they can manage 21 straight successful and exempt days, they figure they have the habit down well enough to stop bothering keeping track. Others shoot for a solid month because it looks so visually compelling on a calendar. Others keep going indefinitely because the expense of keeping track in this way is so low and they feel the motivational benefits outweigh the effort.

I would suggest trying the Habit Traffic Light for at least a solid calendar month instead of just going for a certain number of consecutive successes. That way you use the motivational power of the calendar to its best effect, and you won't be inordinately depressed by a failure that breaks your winning streak. A failure or two in a month still hurts—you'd rather not see those splotches of red—but you can recover more easily when you don't feel you've lost all your previous gains. That sea of green is still there: your failures don't undo your successes.

Looking at it month by month also makes it easier to think about what a good level of compliance would be. I've found it helpful to use an Olympic metaphor as a rule of thumb: 0 failures in a month is gold, 1 is silver, and 2 is bronze—3 or more means better luck next month. I give myself up to two non-weekend S days a month; any more than that count as failures for the purpose of assigning the monthly medal. This Olympic metaphor (I call it *Personal Olympics*) encourages and quantifies success while at the same time tolerating some inevitable imperfection.

If you feel that the Habit Traffic Light adds more complexity than it is worth, skip it. Keeping track even to this minimal degree is an effort, and if you can manage without, then by all means do. I didn't even think of this tool until three years after I started the No S Diet, so

✳ While a paper calendar and colored markers work just fine, you can create a free online Habit Calendar for the No S Diet (and other habits) at www.everydaysystems.com/ habitcal. See page 178 for more details.

it's certainly not necessary. Nonetheless, it does seem to be helpful for many people, and especially if you're having trouble, you might want to consider it.

What If the Diet's Not Working?

Let's say you've taken my advice about putting the scale in perspective and focusing on behavior. Let's say you've even used the Habit Traffic Light and have three months of solid green behind you. And then let's say your occasional sanity check on the scale tells you that even after this good long time, you still haven't lost any weight, maybe you've even gained a few pounds. Well, perspective and all, that's kind of depressing. What should you do?

The first thing is make sure you are assessing the situation correctly. Take the average of several scale measurements over a few days—maybe the initial number was a fluke. Then take a closer look at that calendar: Are there really no red failures in there? If so, how many? How about non-weekend special days? If you have more than two failures or non-weekend special days a month, that might explain the problem. In that case, the next step is obvious: Don't add any new rules, just tighten your compliance around the existing ones, nothing too ruthless, just try to keep the failures plus non-weekend S days to less than three a month.

But what if your behavior really has been perfect, or close to it, and the scale really hasn't budged after all this time? Don't despair. You're still in better shape than before. Before, it was very difficult to know how much you were eating. With the No S Diet, it's easy, because there are far fewer inputs to monitor. You should be able to determine with confidence whether you are in fact eating less. If you're confident you're eating less, great. A little more patience might be all you need to start seeing results.

But what if you feel that you actually are squeezing in a lot of food into the legitimate input opportunities? You're still ahead. Because the No S Diet gives you more than a vague sense that excess is creeping in; it will make it clear *where*. Are there any particular situations, meals, days? I bet you can narrow it down. Shine the spotlight of your attention on those areas. Don't make any grand resolutions up front, just make sure that when you're in a situation in which you tend to overeat, you *notice* it. That attention might be enough by itself to correct the problem without adding any formal rules.

But if necessary, the No S Diet gives you a solid platform from which to take further systematic action. You can build on this foundation of good habits instead of knocking it down and starting from scratch. For example, maybe you need to consider limiting exceptions to once an S day (see page 169), or maybe you need to reclassify some borderline food (like orange juice) as an S food, or maybe you even want to incorporate elements from some other diet plan (see page 167).

But build slowly, or the whole structure will come toppling down under the weight of these new restrictions. You don't want to risk the moderate, sustainable platform you now have with extreme interventions. Remember that for most of us, maintenance *is* progress, the status quo was gaining weight.

If you're feeling impatient and considering more extreme dietary interventions, you're better off looking at the amount of exercise you are getting. Making two moderate efforts—diet *and* exercise—is far safer, easier, and more sustainable than picking just one and making an extreme effort. If *exercise* is synonymous with *torture* in your mind, don't give up on it just yet; it doesn't have to be that bad. And it doesn't take much; it just takes *consistency*. See page 173 for some suggestions on how to use the underlying principles of the No S Diet to incorporate a moderate exercise routine into your life.

Resisting Excuses

Habit takes a while to form; and while it's forming, and your conscious mind is still doing a fair share of the grunt work, that conscious mind is going to come up with an astonishing array of excuses to shirk its duties. The clarity of the No S Diet rules, and their humaneness, are a great defense against this tendency, but the rules are not foolproof. It's important to remind yourself that reinforcements are on the way, that habit will soon start to take over from your conscious mind. But it's also important to have a sense of humor: The best way to dispatch excuses is to laugh at them. I call this *enlightened self-mockery*.

Being fat might be bad, but get over yourself—it's not a tragedy. Sophocles or Euripides never wrote any plays about it. Instead, try to have a sense of humor about your predicament. If you shake your head and laugh at your weaknesses instead of tearfully castigating yourself, your odds of succeeding are going to be dramatically (in both senses of the word) improved. Make this a comedy instead of a tragedy.

But remember, *enlightened* self-mockery—no *Goodfellas*-style "ball busting." In that spirit, I'll close this chapter by poking some good-natured fun at the most common excuses that keep people from succeeding on the No S Diet.

But I'm Genetically Fat!

It's certainly possible to be "genetically fat," but you probably aren't. If you're like most overweight people, it's no mystery why you're fat. You're fat because you eat too much. I don't care whether it's carbs or hydrogenated oils or granola bars, you just eat a lot of it. Maybe you don't metabolize your food quite as efficiently as your skinny neighbor, I'll grant you that (for the sake of argument); but the fact remains, you eat too much. I don't mean to be insulting; I used to eat too much, too. I put it this way because you're never going to lose any weight if you don't assume responsibility for the situation. So get this genes stuff out of your head; it's probably just an excuse, and it certainly won't solve the problem.

According to the Centers for Disease Control and

Prevention (CDC), the obesity rate in the United States has *doubled* since 1980.[3] Rapid mutation? Sorry, folks, evolution doesn't work that fast.

> *Despite obesity having strong genetic determinants, the genetic composition of the population does not change rapidly. Therefore, the large increase in…[obesity] must reflect major changes in non-genetic factors.*[4]

The obesity rate in populations like the Old Order Amish, who have sufficient food and traditional life-styles, is about 4 percent. Ours is over 30 percent. That would seem to indicate that the difference, almost 90 percent of obesity today, is due to behavioral factors (and this assumes that 0 percent of the Amish are obese for *non*genetic reasons).[5]

If you're still convinced that you've been doomed by your genes (you might, after all, be one of those unlucky 4 percent), view this diet as an experiment. If you can stick with it for six months and not lose a significant amount of weight, then you can plead genetics with a clear conscience. And I suspect you'll be at least a somewhat skinnier genetically fat person.

You'll also know with confidence that you are not overeating, and there's something to be said for that even if you don't lose much weight. Immoderate eating, what used to be called gluttony, is an evil even apart from its effects. Sure it makes us fat, but it also puts us out of control. It makes us slaves to our appetite. We feel degraded and unhappy, not so much because of what other people say or think, but because of an *actual* lack of freedom. On the No S Diet, you get back in control. And whatever your body mass index (BMI), that's a much better way to live.

My Coworkers Will Be Offended If I Don't Eat the Goodies They're Always Bringing In!

> *I cannot believe the food that is available at work tempting me all day. Candy, pastries, sweet stuff everywhere. People are always bringing some type of goodies to work. I have trouble saying no, because I don't want to hurt anybody's feelings.*
>
> —CarrieAnn from the
> Nosdiet.com bulletin board

Is your office a veritable dumping ground for sweet treats, a constant source of temptation? The combination of sugar and social pressure can seem overwhelming. But next time your coworkers bring goodies to work, try resisting—just as an experiment. I think you'll be amazed at how little other people care about or even notice what you eat. In most office situations, the food is just lying around; it's anonymous. You really aren't going to hurt anyone's feelings by not eating it.

If everyone around you is convivially indulging and you feel like you're sticking out, grab a mug of black coffee or a glass of water. A drink is the perfect no-calorie social prop. It will give you something to do with your hands; and by consuming something, you'll seem to be joining in the group. See "Old-Fashioned Excuses for Virtue" on page 148 if by some improbable fluke someone does say something.

Be careful not to let social pressure be an excuse for the more basic pressure of animal appetite, which is hard enough to deal with when it's not all tarted up in virtuous clothing. Most of the food people dump at the office isn't even that good—if there is ever a time to be a food snob, this is it. It might be enough to break the spell to simply ask yourself, "If no one cares, and the food isn't even good, why do I feel tempted?"

My Mother-in-Law Will Be Offended If I Don't Eat Multiple Servings of the Special Treat She Made for Me!

Coworkers are one thing. Mothers-in-law are quite another. Most of the time social pressure will not be a real issue; the social unobtrusiveness of the No S Diet is one of its biggest selling points—people are unlikely to even *notice* what you're doing, much less object. However, there are certainly times when you will feel it. In fact, the only thing that ever causes me to slip these days is social pressure like this. You could put me in a room full of the most delicious French pastries, and I wouldn't think of touching them on an N day. But insert a guilt-tripping relative into the room and there might (rarely) be a problem.

Fortunately for most of us, if we're honest with ourselves, these situations are unusual. A simple, "No thanks, it looks delicious, but I'm really full. Can I save it for later?" will almost always do the trick. For those occasions when it doesn't—well, listen to your mother-in-law. No one is perfect; even I cave in on this issue now and then. Domestic tranquility is worth a few extra calories once in a blue moon.

If this is a problem that comes up frequently with particular relatives, I'm afraid you've got no choice but to sit down with them and have a little chat. It might be awkward at first, but because you're asking so little of them (imagine if you were trying to get your mother-in-law to cook low-carb for you instead!) chances are they won't be offended or annoyed; on the contrary, they might even be impressed (especially if they're from an older generation with strong memories of the traditional modes of eating that the No S Diet emulates). What's more, you've left them plenty of scope for unbridled culinary generosity—on S days. Once your relatives understand the system, it's very easy for them to work with it.

I'm Too Stressed-Out to Worry About Diet!

Giving it up when things become stressful is…well, misguided. It'll make you more stressed. I'm not sure if mere logic helps when stress strikes, but it's worth a shot.

Stress is inevitable. It's not a matter of *if*, but *when*. Here are some things you can do to brace yourself for it:

* Keep your focus on a sustainable minimum of compliance instead of one-off heroics. The most important function of each day's behavior is not its physical results but its place in the chain of habit, its role in keeping your habit going. When stress comes, tell yourself, "I just have to make a token effort to keep the habit going. I'm not going to care how big my plates are today, as long as I stick with one per meal. I'm not going to begrudge

myself a glass of milk in the afternoon when I get hungry, as long as there's no cookie with it."

* Sometimes stress will get the better of you no matter how hard you try. Even I—years into these habits and with founder's zeal and all—(very) occasionally allow myself to be pressured into breaking a No S Diet rule. Be honest about these failures, and limit them. One day is regrettable but inevitable. Two in a row is pushing it. And it should never be more than that. Don't beat yourself up, just hit the brakes hard. Marking green, yellow, and red (respectively) for success, exemption, and failure on a Habit Traffic Light calendar helps. Just make sure not to stop marking when you run into a failure; that's the most important thing to mark.

* Remember that the best antidote to stress is routine. I know this is hard to believe when the world seems to be collapsing around you, but in times of stress, routine is *more* important than it usually is, not less. An island of regularity in a sea of chaos gives you a calm, stable base of operations from which to address those other stresses. Lose that island and everything is just drifting.

Stress and craziness seem temporary. But they're really kind of permanent, with intermissions. It's important not to get into the "as soon as things calm down I'll do what I should" mentality because things never stay calm for long, and so if you think that way you'll never do what you should.

I'm an Emotional Eater! When I'm
Depressed, Food Is My Only Comfort

On one level, emotional eating is just an obviously terrible strategy. It not only makes you fat but also it doesn't even work as comfort (for more than a few minutes). And the truth is—and this is what makes it such a difficult problem to deal with—that emotional eating is at least as much about self-punishment as it is about consolation: force-feeding as a kind of self-revenge, a sugar-coated scourge. The mentality behind it is really quite similar to that behind binging and purging; the only difference is the means of discipline: more food instead of less.

It works something like this: You think, "I messed up. I'm trying to lose weight, but I ate a cookie. I feel low and powerless. The only power I feel I can exert is to make myself even lower. So *I'll eat 10 more*." You split yourself into two parts: the punisher and the punished. You identify with the punisher and forget that the punished has anything to do with you; until 10 minutes later, when you come down from your illusory high of self-empowerment and find yourself stuck with your whole fat self again.

It's important to note that the impetus for a bout of emotional eating, the infraction you're seeking to punish, doesn't have to come from something dietary—in fact, it usually doesn't. You could be feeling low and powerless because you had a bad day at the office; a bag of cookies is still an effective means of self-revenge. The fact that it superficially seems like comfort just serves to get it past your "Whoa, that's messed up" radar.

The standard advice for how to deal with emotional

eating is to find other comfort activities that don't involve food. The problem is, as I've pointed out, that emotional eating often isn't really about comfort—on the contrary. So I'm not sure how effective that strategy will be. By all means, have an emergency-response activity lined up when the urge strikes; just keep in mind that the response isn't necessarily about replacing a *comfort*.

Your most important countermeasure is to recognize the self-destructive element of emotional eating. This is bad stuff. Take it seriously. Don't be fooled by the sugar coating: You're not being nice to yourself by indulging; you're being profoundly mean. It isn't misguided tolerance; it's misguided intolerance.

Merely seeing the real problem isn't going to solve it for you, but it's a start. Here are some more practical tips:

* Redirect the self-punishing impulse behind emotional eating so that it fuels something positive. Bad as this impulse is, there is something you can work with here, a redeemable neutral core. With a little bit of planning, you can turn destructive self-punishment into constructive self-discipline. Exercise is great in this respect because let's face it, most of us don't like exercise. So what better form of "self-punishment" than to hit the gym (or equivalent) instead of yourself. Taking a walk works really well for me. It clears my mind and keeps me far from the refrigerator, and I can do it at a moment's notice; it doesn't require any special planning or equipment. And it's pleasant, once I get over the hurdle of deciding to do it—an *actual* comfort.

* Because you've identified emotional eating as a primary problem, be superstrict about not doing it. Instead of an excuse, it should be an anti-excuse: forbidden to the highest degree, a self-hate crime. You need habit on your side—and quickly—to beat this problem; strictness is the key to enlisting it.

* I hate to pass the buck, but being overweight is rarely the sole or primary cause of the depression that fuels emotional eating. Try to identify the other nondiet problems that are getting you down and break off tractable chunks to deal with as you can. The smaller the chunks, the easier they are to deal with. If you're left with chunks that still seem overwhelming, it might be time to seek professional help (probably not a bad idea in any case).

But I Have Uncontrollable Cravings!
I Can't Resist Them! I'm Addicted to Food!
There are people in this world who are genuine addicts. Put them in a certain trigger situation, and they cannot help but act in a certain (usually bad) way. But for most of us, the word *addiction* is far too simplistic. It's both more accurate and more effective to speak in terms of *habit*.

I've spent most of this chapter talking up habit already; here I'd just like to briefly compare it to addiction. Both of these terms describe powerful, irrational forces—mental associations that push you to act in certain ways under certain conditions. But addiction describes a force that is irresistible, unchangeable, and bad; the best you can hope for is to avoid trigger situations. Habits, though perhaps very powerful, can be opposed. They can be changed. And, most importantly, they can be good as well as bad.

So be very careful when you use words like *addiction* and *craving*. By using terminology like this, you frame the problem in a way that suggests that it is hopeless, and that can be a self-fulfilling prophecy. If you think in terms of habit instead, you turn your problem into a powerful potential ally.

But I Want an Excuse, Not a Solution!

It sounds crazy, but a lot of people would rather have an impressive excuse than accept responsibility for finding a solution. They'd prefer to stay fat and blame McDonald's or refined carbohydrates or hydrogenated vegetable oil or their lousy genes or anyone and anything but themselves. I'm not saying these things aren't factors, but they are not the decisive factor. The decisive factor is just that: human decision.

Don't be afraid of responsibility. Responsibility can be liberating. If it's your fault, then chances are you can fix it. If it's not your fault, then you probably can't. Would you really prefer that a problem be insoluble than have to work to fix it? And yes, thinking makes it so.

People have done all kinds of remarkable things because they thought they could. People routinely fail to do quite ordinary things because they assume they can't.

Health aside, I'm amazed at how many people prefer to trade their sense of free will and human dignity for carte blanche to fail. It's like Esau selling his divine

✳ Don't be afraid of responsibility. Responsibility can be liberating.

birthright for a mess of pottage, choosing to be a slave because it is easier than being free. If you're one of those people, keep searching; this diet isn't for you.

I've Been on the Diet a Whole Week and I'm Not Skinny Yet!

Don't wig out if you don't lose 10 pounds the first day. This is a marathon, not a sprint. Progress is slow, but maintainable. It's going to take a while but it's also going to last a while—your whole life. Don't sabotage your efforts with quick-fix expectations.

But I Know Someone Who Lost a Ton of Weight on Some Other Diet!

Do you have friends or neighbors who can't stop bragging about the weight they lost on the latest fad diet? Good for them. They're lucky. Most people who tried that diet failed (according to the U.S. Food and Drug Administration, 95 percent of dieters fail to stick with their plans[6]). And hey, though I wish them the best, there's still plenty of time left for that: a whole lifetime.

It's a little nightmarish to imagine spending your whole life on most diets. Think about it. If your goal is a nightmare, how can you possibly succeed? If you can't even imagine it, how on earth are you going to do it? Why would you even want to?

Conventional diets aren't ineffective in an abstract, biochemical sense. If you stick with one, you'll probably lose weight. They're just really unpleasant and difficult to adhere to long term, so you almost certainly won't. Occasionally, someone does manage to stick it out for a few months or years. But the vast majority of people don't. So put your diet envy aside and go with what not only works (the easy part) but also allows you pleasant dreams for the future.

Old-Fashioned Excuses for Virtue

We're all too familiar with excuses for failure (genes, cravings, stress, depression, social pressure), but there are plenty of excuses for success in the repertoire too. They're a little dusty but very compelling. Keep them in mind for social situations in which people are consuming S foods all around you (seconds, snacks, sweets).

If someone offers you seconds, say, "No thanks, I've had plenty. I'm full." If someone offers you snacks or sweets between meals, say, "No thanks. I don't want to spoil my appetite."

Remember how worried our mothers used to be about us "spoiling our appetites"? We used to hear phrases like that all the time. They're almost quaint and nostalgic now. Let's bring them back and make excuses something positive. If people smirk, they'd better be skinny.

7

Beyond the No S Diet

Beyond Moderation

Well, we're at the last chapter of the book already, and I've barely mentioned several topics that make up the bulk of most other diet books: nutrition, specific kinds of foods, and—above all—recipes. Why have I neglected these? Not because they aren't interesting or important but because they are *separate issues*. I couldn't do any of them justice by lumping them all together as most diet books do.

The No S Diet solves one problem very well, that of moderating excessive eating. It couldn't do this nearly as well if it were simultaneously aiming at all these other side problems. Moderation is a big enough problem for one system; going beyond that would add unacceptable complexity. Because it may not be immediately clear to you how all these diet-related issues are separate, I'll now say a few words about some of the chief contenders, along with justifications for why I didn't include more extensive treatment of them in this book.

Are There Any No S Diet Recipes?

Recipes make great page fillers, which is why other diet books are jam-packed with them. But have you ever eaten a meal cooked from a recipe in a diet book? My experience has been that they're pretty disgusting. Diet books tend not to be written by people who actually like to eat. I do like to eat—far too much to give that subject short shrift here. I decided I'd rather save you time and money and an upset stomach by leaving recipes out.

Besides, the No S Diet isn't about *what* so much as *when* you eat. You can eat anything you want—at the right time. So use your normal cookbook. It's No S Diet approved.

Preparing recipes from *any* cookbook is likely to help you lose weight over the long run. Why? Because when you cook, you eat in. And when you eat in, you'll usually eat less food than you would at restaurants, with their increasingly enormous portions. Normal cookbooks, cookbooks that make no pretensions to healthfulness, are much better than diet cookbooks in terms of weight management because their recipes taste good enough that you'll actually make them. Healthy recipes that you never make or avoid eating because you don't enjoy them are *bad* for your health because they keep you from cooking and prompt you to eat out—to *overeat* out—instead.

Please Tell Me *Exactly* Every Single Food I Can and Can't Eat!

Sorry, I don't have the time to list foods for you. And it's really not necessary. *Sweet* as I've defined it means "very sweet." If you have to wonder, it's probably okay.

Just about every diet guru publishes a list of permitted and forbidden foods. And those books are bestsellers. People buy millions of copies of these lists. I am utterly baffled by this phenomenon.

I'm baffled because it's so hopeless an enterprise; there are, for all practical purposes, an infinite number of foods. I'm baffled because the things that wind up being forbidden are often so absurd: beets, for example. I guarantee you, no one ever got fat from eating beets. If you see a fat person eating beets, that's not why he's fat. Carrots, formerly the quintessential health food—something people used to carry around in plastic bags as a healthy snack—are now vegetable non grata (high glycemic index, apparently). But most of all, I'm baffled that anyone really imagines they will play scavenger hunt at the supermarket for more than a month or two. It shows an utter ignorance of human psychology.

And yet, as I mentioned, people buy millions of copies of these books of lists. They must get something out of it. Maybe they get an insider-information rush out of reading these oddball restrictions and think, "Whew, glad I know about beets. They would have killed me for sure." What these people don't get is any thinner. The lists may be good for a thrill, but they are psychological suicide as far as losing weight is concerned. Who is really going to run around a supermarket with a book in hand? For a week, maybe. For a month, maybe. But that's it. At that point most of us would feel justly overwhelmed. But maybe that's all some people ever wanted.

The forbidden-food diets, with their hidden-culprit-in-your-pantry theories, are dangerous distractions. They keep you from seeing and confronting the real problem. This isn't *Murder, She Wrote*. It's not the mousy school-marm whom no one ever suspected who winds up having "dunnit." It's a brazen attack in broad daylight. The culprit isn't some problem food you haven't thought of. Take a look in the mirror. The responsible party is staring right at you.

Still want to count carbs, calories, fat, or whatever after all this? Save your money and look at the U.S. Department of Agriculture's nutrient data library at www.ars.usda.gov. Endlessly fascinating, if you have nothing better to do. Those bestselling guru lists are just less accurate and comprehensive versions of the free one from the government.

Can You at Least Tell Me What to Eat for *Breakfast*?

Lunch and diner, everyone seems to be able to figure out; but judging by the volume of Nosdiet.com bulletin board posts on the subject, there are an awful lot of sugary breakfast eaters out there. If you're one of these and are having trouble imagining other possibilities, here are a few ideas to get you started:

* Grown-up cold cereal, like muesli and granola. Remember that *some* sugar is okay. If you're worried about the amount of sugar in your granola (these cereals can be very sweet) cut it 50/50 with an unsweetened cereal like Grape-Nuts or (my favorite) Ezekiel 4:9 (Grape-Nuts with divine mandate).
* Hot cereal, like oatmeal or Cream of Wheat
* Eggs (with bacon, ham, whatever)
* Bread, toast, English muffin with cheese, peanut butter, or cold cuts
* Dinner leftovers. Diced and reheated with a bit of egg, bacon, or cheese in a skillet, anything becomes breakfasty.

And of course, remember to enjoy plenty of fresh fruit with all of the above.

Sound like a big adjustment? I think you'll be surprised at how easy it is. And don't worry, you can still have your beloved pancakes, waffles, Pop-Tarts, or sugar cereal come the weekend. You don't really need to eat them *every* day, do you?

Is That Really All You're Going to Say About Nutrition?

As I mentioned in Chapter 1, the No S Diet doesn't explicitly address nutrition—beyond the issue of simple excess, which is probably the single most pressing nutritional problem confronting First Worlders today. But it does address the broader subject of nutrition *implicitly*, as a kind of side effect. By limiting your input opportunities to single-plate meals, you put a spotlight not just on excess but on your other nutritional choices as well.

When you have to choose between an apple and a pile of chips because only one will fit on your plate, both the cost of that pile of chips and the value of the apple become clear. The limited input opportunities of the No S Diet mean you have to choose between options; you can't have everything. By making poor nutritional choices obvious, you are forced to *see* the other tradeoffs you are making. Some of the time, the pleasure you get from those chips might be worth it to you. But much of the time, most of the time, if the choice is presented this clearly, it won't. So without any explicit rules governing the situation, you'll eat more apples and fewer chips. It won't happen this way all the time, but it will happen enough. And that's really all you need.

Nutrition is simultaneously a very complex problem, when you look at it from a descriptive, biochemical perspective, and a very simple one, when you look at it from the perspective of an individual who wants to eat right. The truth is, unless you have some special medical condition, you probably already know all you need to know. If

✳ Micheal Pollan, author of *The Omnivore's Dilemma,* puts it even more succinctly: "Eat food. Not too much. Mostly plants. That, more or less, is the short answer to the supposedly incredibly complicated and confusing question of what we humans should eat in order to be maximally healthy."[1]

not, here it goes: (1) Eat less. (2) Eat a greater *percentage* of fresh fruits, vegetables, and whole grains. (3) Reduce your intake of highly processed foods correspondingly.

Finding it hard to translate that simple advice into action? There's nothing like the spotlight of single-plate meals to force the issue.

So don't worry about blueberries versus pomegranates versus the current trendy superfood; hedge your bets and eat a variety of foods. If you insist on making nutrition more complex than this, all you're doing is providing a smoke screen for excess to creep in. You'll wind up using nutrition as an excuse to overeat. You'll be confused and distracted from the main issue of eating less. Unscrupulous marketers will compound the problem (*low fat, low sugar, rich in omega-3s* are all euphemisms for "eat more!"). You'll force yourself to eat worse-tasting food in the name of nutrition and then take revenge by binging on yummy junk.

In *Mindless Eating*, Brian Wansink describes a curious phenomenon: When products are marketed as healthy, people eat more of them because they think, "Hey, it's healthy." They'll even go on to eat more of some obviously unhealthy food because they think, "Hey, I just ate something healthy, I've got virtue to burn." They feel somehow blessed by this contact with the healthy food. Wansink calls this the "health halo" effect. And it's obviously very unhealthy. Don't fall for it.[2]

If despite all these warnings you feel the need to take a systematic approach toward nutrition as well, be my guest. The No S Diet is compatible with pretty much every other diet plan I've come across. You can be a No S vegan if you want. You could even do a No S Diet plus Atkins or a No S Diet plus the Zone, if you want to hedge your weight-loss bets (though I think it's becoming increasingly clear these last two examples are emphatically *not* going to help you in the nutrition department, if at all).

What About Carbs?

As I pointed out in Chapter 3, sweets are largely sugar, and sugar is a carb—the most nutritionally undesirable carb there is. So because the No S Diet reduces your sugar intake, it is technically a kind of low-carb diet. But it doesn't restrict carbs beyond sweets because that would be unnecessary, unpleasant, and possibly dangerous.

I'm not saying it's protein and fat that make us fat, that if you twiddle the percentages a bit you'll come out all right. What I'm saying is that it clearly doesn't look as if carbs in and of themselves are the culprit for our obesity epidemic, because, as I discussed in Chapter 3, we actually eat relatively less of them compared to the skinny rest of the world and our own skinny ancestors. If people who eat a much higher percentage of carbs than we do are thin, then it seems unlikely that their diet is what made us fat. The obvious culprit is the fact that we eat *absolutely* more of everything: more fat, more protein, and more carbs. And that's the culprit that the No S Diet focuses on.

What About Fat?

I don't want to seem like I'm coming down as pro-fat in the carbs-versus-fat debate, either. I think the evidence strongly suggests that too much fat is bad for you. But I also think that much (if not most) of the excessive fat people consume is in the form of snack foods and sweets, which are restricted by the No S Diet. (They also tend to contain the worst kinds of fat, those notorious highly processed trans-fats.) So while the No S Diet does not address fat explicitly, it does so as a kind of side effect.

The reason I don't address fat explicitly, besides the fact that the side-effect restriction seems just fine to me, is that dietary fat is a more complex issue than sugar. There are good fats and bad fats, and it's often less clear which foods are high in fat (whereas sugar tends to jump right out at you). Simplicity and clarity are important. If you had a complicated diet that was 100 percent in sync with the latest nutritional research and covered every theoretical base, it wouldn't do you any good if you couldn't stick with it (never mind that the latest nutritional research is a rapidly moving target). Zero percent of one hundred is zero. An 80 percent solution that you can actually stick with is infinitely preferable to that.

What About Junk Food?

You can technically eat junk food on the No S Diet. But because you can't snack, and most junk food is snack food, you'll probably eat much less of it. And the spotlight that having limited input opportunities puts on your meals means you won't want to waste them on junk. I know this seems hard to believe now, but once you get a few weeks of good mealing habits under your belt, that pile of Cheetos on your plate just won't seem right.

So the No S Diet doesn't directly address the issue of junk food, not because it isn't an important issue, but because it is adequately addressed as a side effect. If you find that in your case that's not good enough, then you might want to take additional measures. But I very much doubt that this will be necessary, so I'm not going to get into it here. Beware unnecessary prohibitions. If you inflict too many rules on yourself, you run the risk of provoking a powerful and destructive reaction.

What About Fast Food?

Fast food is a little trickier than junk food because fast food is (mostly) meal food—highly processed, highly caloric, nutritionally vacuous meal food. It's bad stuff, but bad stuff that you are technically allowed to eat on the No S Diet.

Some people have lost weight on the No S Diet while eating many of their meals in fast-food joints, but obviously this isn't the best idea. I eat fast food occasionally and don't worry about it. But if you're doing it regularly, you'll have a much easier time losing weight if you cut down. As I mentioned in Chapter 4, fast-food restaurants use the very psychology that the No S Diet uses to help you eyeball excess *against* you. They know that you'll be embarrassed to order two fries or two colas, so they just roll those two portions' worth into one mega-portion—and charge accordingly. You can navigate around these tricks by ordering carefully; but be honest with yourself, are you really going to? Better play it safe by keeping your distance.

There is always a danger in adding extra dietary rules, and I don't think extra rules are the solution to a fast-food problem, if you have one. Stick with the No S Diet rules as a baseline, and come up with some positive alternatives to fast food, some *Intelligent Dietary Defaults* for situations in which you'd otherwise opt for McDonald's.

Intelligent Dietary Defaults

The concept of *intelligent defaults* comes from the computer world. Default settings enable users of a computer program to work with it without having to explicitly state all their preferences. The programmers make some guesses about what most users would like and code the program to behave that way unless the user specifies otherwise. If the default is a good guess, then it's "intelligent." Users can override the defaults if they want to, but they usually won't because the settings make a good amount of sense for most people in most cases. Just imagine if you had to explicitly set every possible preference in order to use a complex program like Microsoft Word; it would take you hours or days just to get to the point at which you could start writing a simple thank-you note.

It's funny that this concept of defaults originated with computers and not in human psychology, because although it's possible to imagine a computer program without defaults—a (very irritating) program that requires you to explicitly set every possible preference before using it—it's not possible to imagine a human being without default behaviors: unthinking, automatic responses to certain kinds of situations. And, unfortunately, many of those human defaults (particularly regarding diet) are not at all intelligent.

When we actively think, most of us are capable of making good dietary decisions. But most of the time, when we're being harried by a million external pressures, diet is pretty low on our list of concerns, and we unthinkingly reach for whatever is most convenient, which tends to be highly processed, highly caloric junk food. This unthinking reflex eating is more or less a fact of life. We can try to eat more mindfully, but to some extent it's hopeless. A smarter thing to do would be to arrange it so that the convenient thing we unthinkingly reach for—the default—is reasonably healthy. Making the default smart doesn't deprive us of any freedom; we're still just as free to override the default. It just makes the choice of *not* choosing (which most people, sadly, opt for) a better one. There is always a default; why not make it a good one?

The key to coming up with good dietary defaults is to accept the fact that you're going to have to compromise between competing concerns. The healthiest

There is always a default; why not make it a good one?

things are in many cases not terribly convenient or cheap enough for routine consumption, or you may find them utterly disgusting. Convenience, price, and taste are goods that also need to be weighed in the balance. The other key is not to force yourself into eating this stuff *every* time. Default doesn't mean obligatory. It just means what you do when nothing better comes along. And better doesn't have to be healthier; it can be socially better, like participating in a group lunch, or gastronomically better, like having a delicious meal at a fancy restaurant. The default is for when you are in an unthinking rush, which is a lot of the time for most of us. Changing your behavior in these situations is enough to make a significant difference.

But don't go overboard. There's a saying in the computer world that "premature optimization is the root of all evil." In other words, don't start optimizing until you have a good sense of the problem, until your program more or less does what it's supposed to, or you're going to waste massive effort on relatively insignificant details. Get to good before you worry about better or best. In the case of diet, the issue of excessive eating, pure and simple, is the giant heart of the problem, and you shouldn't let fine-tuning distract you from that. So make sure you have the basics of the No S Diet down first, then (maybe) consider adding optimizations like intelligent defaults.

Here's one example of an Intelligent Dietary Default that's been working well for me for years: I call it *Optimize Your Oatmeal*. While it's unlikely that you'll want to adopt this *exact* default (dietary defaults, like tastes, tend to be very personal), the thought processes behind it might be useful when coming up with your own.

Here's the problem: If I don't prepare my lunch in advance, the default thing would be to go to a fast-food joint in close proximity to my office—or, worse, to grab a bag of junk from the vending machine. But preparing lunch in advance can take an awful lot of forethought, and I've never consistently been able to pull that off. The solution: A zero-forethought, cheap, convenient, and reasonably healthy alternative—oatmeal for lunch.

As for the name, *optimize* is another computer term. On one level, its meaning is obvious, "to make better." But it also has the connotation of "optimize for what?" There's this implied question. And there's a whole science of optimization that has to do with managing and balancing competing concerns. I think Optimize Your Oatmeal does this rather brilliantly.

Here's what I do: I eat rolled oats, not instant, but the way I prepare it is more or less instantaneous. I pour some oatmeal in a bowl, mix in some kind of nuts, some kind of seeds, and some kind of dried fruits. Then I go to the hot-water spigot by the coffee machine and cover it with hot water. By the time I'm back at my desk it's ready to eat. The oats don't really cook much. They just get sort of warmed up and a little softened. I like them this way. It gives me something to bite on. In fact, the kind of oatmeal I buy, Old Wessex Scottish-

Style Porridge Oats, advertises itself (quite accurately) as "chewy, chewy, chewy" on the box. And I buy it for that reason. Other varieties of rolled oats don't necessarily stay chewy enough for me, even with this very mild warming up.

The first advantage of preparing oatmeal like this is that it is quick. Most of the prep time consists of walking back and forth from my desk to the hot-water spigot. It's so quick, in fact, that I have a good 45 minutes left over on my lunch break to walk around outside and get some exercise.

It's convenient. I don't have to store anything in the communal refrigerator at work (or get into perpetual battles about who made what mess or who took whose lunch). All the ingredients are dry; I can buy them way in advance and store them in a drawer in my desk. I don't even have to use the communal microwave, because all I need for heat is the hot-water spigot. The reason I eat this for lunch at work rather than home is because at home I've got all these great resources: a non-nasty communal refrigerator, an oven, and pots and pans. I might as well save the resource-intensive cooking (which I do enjoy) for when I actually have these resources, and resort to the quick convenient stuff when I don't.

It's socially flexible. If your coworkers unexpectedly invite you out to lunch, you can skip your oatmeal and join them without having to worry about your food going bad. Unlike perishable bagged lunches, these ingredients will keep.

Oatmeal is cheap. They feed this stuff to horses. It's cheaper than cat food. Yes, the dried fruits and nuts can add up, but we're still talking less than a dollar a day for lunch.

Oatmeal is healthy. It's whole grain. It's relatively unprocessed. I guess the steel-cut kind would be better, but it loses too many points on convenience. Dried fruit may not be as healthy as fresh fruit; but hey, it's still fruit. And I have plenty of fresh fruit with other meals.

Finally, oatmeal is filling. It's like eating cement. The first time you prepare oatmeal like this you won't be able to finish it because you'll have made too much. This is particularly relevant for No S Dieters, because if you eat oatmeal for lunch, you will *not* be hungry until dinnertime.

This is just one example of many possible Intelligent Dietary Defaults. The point I'm trying to make here is not to convince you to eat oatmeal (although that wouldn't be a *bad* thing). I just want to provide you with one very concrete, in-depth example of some of the factors to consider when coming up with your own, personalized dietary defaults.

Here are a few more quick ideas to inspire you:

* B.Y.O.S. (Bring Your Own Sugar). Instead of buying presweetened yogurt, cereal, or peanut butter, buy the unsweetened kind and add your own. Don't put a hard limit on how much you can put in, just observe; that observation by itself will provide an effective limit. I don't care how sweet you like it, there's no way you're going to watch yourself spoon in as much sugar as the manufacturer would invisibly have done for you. After two, three, four

spoonfuls you'll be too embarrassed to continue adding more, and you'll probably find that it tastes just fine. Remember that the no sweets rule does allow you to eat some sugar, so this is completely legitimate. It's another example of how merely forcing yourself to *see* excess can be an effective way of limiting it.

* Fruit shrine. Increased visibility can work both ways. We've talked about how it can discourage you from eating bad stuff, but it can also *encourage* you to eat (relatively) more healthy foods. One way of doing this is to always keep a prominently visible plate of fresh fruit on your table. By not hiding your fruit out of sight, out of mind, deep in the bowels of your refrigerator, you'll remember to reach for it instead of less healthy stuff, and it will be obvious when your supply needs replenishing. If you're worried about your fruit shrine rotting at room temperature, there's a positive side to that: incentive to buy more frequently and fresher (and fresher means healthier) instead of hoarding in bulk. Plus you'll have plenty of time to see what's turning overripe since it's all out in the open. I find I've been throwing away a lot less fruit since I've been practicing this technique. Last but not least, unrefrigerated fruit tastes better—really, try it.

* Black bread breakfast. A company called Mestemacher makes hard-core bricks of whole grain black bread that have more fiber than a tree; and they're not bad tasting once you get used to them. Inspired

by Westphalian pumpernickel, this isn't some con-
coction out of a lab but a traditional food that
just happens to be healthy and convenient. It's
dense, long lasting, quick to prepare, ridiculously
good for you, and *filling*. A single slice, toasted or
untoasted, makes a great European-style open-
face sandwich topped with cheese, peanut butter, or Schinken (Westphalian prosciutto). Keep a
brick of Mestemacher around and you'll never be
at a loss for what to eat for breakfast—and you
won't get hungry until lunch. Beats the pants off
a Pop-Tart.

* Whole (week) grains. As anyone who cooks knows,
  starches tend take the longest time to prepare of
  any dinner component, and whole grain starches
  take the longest of all. Most of us know we should
  eat more whole grains, but we can't spare the 45 to
  60 minutes they take to prepare from scratch every
  night. The solution? Make a big pot of a whole
  grain starch like brown rice over the weekend when
  you have a bit more time, then reheat portions of it
  as your dinner starch during the week. You could
  even freeze some for longer-term storage. While
  you don't have to resort to it every night, it's a great
  option to have if you're running late and would
  otherwise reach for highly processed convenience
  food instead.

I could go on and on, but remember: Premature
optimization is the root of all evil. While it's helpful to
know that you can build on the foundation provided

by the No S Diet with strategies like these, it's important to keep your focus on the foundation itself.

Combining the No S Diet
with Other Diets

While the No S Diet should be enough all by itself to manage your weight (even without the optimizations described earlier in this chapter), it is accommodating and unobtrusive enough that you could combine it with another diet if you want to hedge your weight-loss bets, want to take a systematic approach to specific nutritional issues, or have religious or ethical dietary considerations such as vegetarianism or keeping kosher. I'd like to emphasize that this isn't necessary, and if you're not committed to something else already I'd strongly caution against loading yourself up with extra rules all at once. But it is possible. People on the Nosdiet.com bulletin board have reported combining it with various types of low-carb plans, the Shangri-La Diet, vegetarianism, and more.

Modifying/Personalizing
the No S Diet

One of the reasons it is so easy for me to stick with the No S Diet is because I invented it. Founder's zeal is a powerful motivator; when it's your brainchild rather than someone else's, you're more profoundly invested in it. So if you're tempted to modify the No S Diet around the edges or to use it as a point of inspiration for a whole new system of your own, you have my blessing and encouragement; and the mere fact that you invented all or part of it will make you more likely to succeed.

That being said, do be careful. The downside of self-made systems is that you feel fewer compunctions about modifying them at the spur of the moment. It's also not trivial to come up with humane shortcuts to caloric restriction; your home brew may not wind up tasting so good, even to you, and it might even wind up toxic. There are always tradeoffs, and they're not always obvious.

The most promising openings for change would be if you have some special routine or situation in your life that might either clash with or actively support good eating behaviors, that you'd like to systematically take into account, so your new habits use this existing structure rather than fighting against it. For example, some people on the Nosdiet.com bulletin board limit their weekly S days to the Sabbath instead of the weekend. That leverages the strength of their religious conviction; preserves the S consonance; cuts out a few more calories; and, if you celebrate sundown to sundown, can be simply a matter of convenience. The downside is that it might be overambitious: Reducing your S days by close to 50 percent might be unsustainably hard and unpleasant.

Another example is if you work weekends. You might want to move your exempt days to match the days you have off from work. There are downsides to this, too (see page 106).

Yet another example is to legitimize snacking on raw fruits and vegetables. People have done this, quite successfully; but it does introduce new dangers that you should be aware of. As snacks go, raw fruits and vegetables are certainly better than the alternatives, but there is the danger that then you feel the right to let your meals decline in quality because you're making up with healthy fruits in between. Your meals will then become more caloric and less nutritious without bulky, healthy fruit to crowd out denser stuff. And then, of course, there is the simple danger of controlling the habit of eating between meals, a habit that might not always be content with mere fruit. If you feel you can navigate this danger, fantastic, but be aware of it.

On the No S website, I've often inserted a parenthetical *sometimes* into the exception part of the No S formula, making it read: "Except (sometimes) on days that start with S." The *sometimes* isn't logically necessary (of course you shouldn't eat snacks, sweets, and seconds *all* the time on S days!) so in the interest of succinctness I left it out of the "canonical" version. But an explicit *sometimes* can be a helpful reminder, so by all means reinsert it if you think mere logic isn't going to do it for you.

Building on this apocryphal *sometimes*, a further No S Diet extension that has been tossed around is to interpret it as meaning "once" (or some similarly small number), if excessive S days are causing problems and you really think you can pull it off. The way this would work is that on every S day you get only *one* exception from the rules, one sweet or one second or one snack—say, popcorn at the movies *or* an ice cream cone after dinner *or* a generous wedge of carrot cake. I would be very hesitant to add this restriction because I think it's important to keep S days as free as possible, but it is a pretty natural extension to the basic No S Diet system if, having weighed all these factors, you still feel you need a little more rigor. But if you do this, be sure to give yourself *some* kind of reward: Whether or not you make it the maximum, "once" should be the minimum.

I could go on, but I don't want to preempt your creativity by attempting to exhaust every possible alternative here. And a degree of personalization is built right into the No S Diet. No one is likely to have exactly the same special days (holidays and vacation days) as you. No one is likely to have problems with the same borderline foods as you, to make the same calls about which of these should be considered sweets. By your choices in these areas, you put a very personal stamp on your version of the No S Diet. It might not be enough personalization for you to feel artistic pride in your creation, but it should be enough for you to feel very comfortable in something that's been sized just for you, like a custom-tailored suit.

Can I Do a "Some S" Diet?

You can do whatever you want with the No S Diet; I'm not going to excommunicate you. But doing a watered-down "some S" version of the diet probably isn't going to be very effective. The thing about a moderate system like the No S Diet is that you actually have to follow it systematically. Because you're cutting off only a bit around the edges, there's not the same leeway of excess that an extreme system will give you. The No S Diet has exceptions built right in, so you don't want to add too many more. The plan isn't that hard. Try doing it strictly for three weeks; that's about how long it takes to form a habit. You'll be surprised.

That being said, the S's don't depend on each other. Each makes sense on its own, and each should be helpful on its own. Do what's possible and necessary for you. Dieting in a "half-essed" manner, as one bulletin-board correspondent put it, can have wholly satisfying results, as long as you're *clear* about which half (or third) you're doing and are no less diligent in sticking to it.

I've often thought that gradually progressing to one S at a time might be a good way to become a full No S Dieter. For example, start with *no sweets* for a week, then add *no seconds* the next week, and then move on to *no snacks* the next week (or go even more slowly and give each S the full magic-habit-building 21 days). That way you could build willpower and habit in incremental, easy-to-achieve baby steps. But I should warn you that, logical as this sounds, I'm not aware that anyone has successfully done it. I think the trouble is that even the full No S Diet is slow in terms of yielding measurable results, and lack of patience is an even bigger problem for most people than lack of short-term willpower.

I Can Think of Other Things That Start with S

Snacks, *sweets*, and *seconds* are not the only dietary dangers that start with the letter S, and you might be tempted to extend the No S Diet framework to take them into account. But be careful: Extra restrictions, no matter how cute, mean extra complexity, extra effort, and extra risk for the whole project.

If you think you can handle these risks, here are some additional S's that have been suggested on the Nosdiet.com bulletin board:

* Soda. Technically already a sugar S, but some people can use the extra reminder.
* Supersizes. No one really needs these and fast-food junkies especially should watch out for them.
* Starch. Not a popular substance with diet gurus, but as I've already mentioned, unless you have special medical issues, it seems to me that drastically reducing starch is excessive and unmaintainable.

Beyond Diet

The underlying principles of the No S Diet can be applied to other behaviors that you might want to change. This could be the result of a conscious, deliberate process; but some of it might happen without your even realizing it. In the next few sections I will discuss some examples of both.

Are There Any Side Effects?

I've already mentioned some of the purely nutritional side effects of the No S Diet: Without explicitly addressing these issues, you'll consume fewer refined carbs, fewer trans-fats, and relatively more nutrient-dense food. But there are side effects that go beyond diet altogether.

By setting your willpower up to succeed, and suc-

✳ Willpower is like a muscle; doing the No S Diet is like working that muscle out with 50 pushups every morning.

ceeding a little bit every day, you build up general-purpose willpower. Willpower is like a muscle; doing the No S Diet is like working that muscle out with 50 pushups every morning. Once your No S habit is firmly in place, you can reallocate that general-purpose willpower to other tasks.

Contrast this with the effects of the repeated failures of willpower associated with mainstream yo-yo dieting, which won't just leave you fat but less fit to do *anything* else.

On the No S Diet, you will also start to enjoy food again, instead of merely obsessing over it. It's sad how many overweight people don't even enjoy all that food they eat. They hate it, both for making them fat and, if they're dieting, for all the intellectual work it represents (counting calories, and so on). The No S Diet doesn't just get you thin, it makes food *food* again, instead of the mere quantity that other diets make it.

What About Exercise?

Of course you should exercise. Diet can't substitute for that. You need to do both. While it's possible to get lean by focusing on just one side of the equation, it's much easier and more sustainable to adjust a bit on both the input and the output ends at the same time. Make two moderate efforts rather than one extreme effort.

Burning calories, building muscle—that's easy. The hard part is sticking to a routine. It's really the same kind of problem as the diet: not a *physiological* one, when you get down to it, but a *psychological* one. Almost any exercise program will get you in shape, *if you stick with it*. But the vast majority of people don't. So forget about muscular efficiency and keep your efforts focused on identifying a program you can actually adhere to over time.

Many of the principles behind the No S Diet will be helpful in coming up with an exercise routine like this:

* Keep the emphasis on *a regular and sustainable minimum of compliance* rather than heroic efforts. It doesn't take much to get into great shape, as long as you do it consistently. I find it helpful to focus on a specific and small amount of exercise *time* rather than any particular kind of exercise (I do 14 minutes; but, obviously, this is a somewhat arbitrary number). Focusing on the time means I'm never in a situation in which I can't do my workout because I'm lacking some special equipment, and I can change the kind of exercise I do without disrupting my schedule. As long as I have 14 minutes, and my hands aren't literally tied behind my back, I have no excuse not to work out. If I'm at home, I'll use my home workout gear. If I'm traveling, I'll do pushups and squats. As with the No S Diet, I make the "minimum equal the maximum": I never work out longer than my allotted time, even if I'm feeling unusually gung-ho, because I don't want to risk my consistent, regu-

lar efforts by overdoing it and burning out. There is a great range of workouts you can get in even just a few minutes. Short workouts can be intense. See how many consecutive minutes of pushups or squats you can do if you don't believe me. But if you're not feeling so pumped-up on a given day, you can take a more leisurely 14 minutes. By doing the time, even at a more relaxed pace, you keep the habit going. And long term, that is going to get you fit. A *timer* is probably the single best piece of exercise equipment you can buy.

* Look for *behaviors that are natural*, that people used to perform in the course of their ordinary daily activities; such behaviors will be easier to turn into unconscious habit. They'll be more fun and interesting than going through the contrived motions of the gym—and that means you'll be more likely to convince yourself to keep doing them. Best of all are movements you can apply to some useful task, like walking or gardening. But routines that mimic potentially useful movements are good, too, like my manual-labor-imitating sledgehammer workout that I've called *Shovelglove* (see www.shovelglove.com).

* Look for *clear rules around when you should exercise* and when you can take off with a clear conscience (the division between N days and S days can be a very natural, helpful structure here). You never want to catch yourself wondering whether you have to exercise on a given day; if you wonder, you won't.

* Make your exercise as *unobtrusive* as possible, so there is a minimum of conflict between it and the rest of your life. A short, simple routine you can do in your living room is vastly preferable to a monster high-tech workout at the gym that also requires a 40-minute commute. A locomotive exercise like walking or biking or taking the stairs whenever possible that actually gets you somewhere you have to go is best of all; it can take no extra time and, depending on traffic conditions, it might even *save* you time.

* *Measure your progress by behavior, not by results.* Don't focus on how many pounds you can lift or miles you can run, but on Days on Habit, days on which you met your clearly defined minimum level of behavioral compliance (that is, days on which you did your allotted time). The Habit Traffic Light I described in Chapter 6 can be a great tool for building exercise habits as well. Force yourself to mark off every day you exercise in green, every day you don't in red, and exempt days in yellow, and soon your exercise routine will be almost automatic.

If you're having trouble figuring out precisely what exercise to do, consider starting with walking. If you feel walking is too, well, pedestrian, get over it. Healthwise, it's the best long-term exercise you can do and the only consistently useful or interesting one. See my www.urbanranger.com website if you need additional inspiration.

Beyond This Book

I've packed (and now unpacked) a whole book's worth of meaning into the dozen-odd words on the cover. Dense stuff, this formula! And there's more: a whole online community.

Is There a *Free* Internet Support Group?

The Internet is where the No S Diet got started, and a thriving group of dieters still gather at Nosdiet .com. At the time of this writing, there are well over 1,000 registered bulletin board users and more than 25,000 messages.

What are all these messages about? Mostly people ask questions and get prompt, courteous answers from a range of perspectives. I pipe in when I can, but sometimes it's more helpful to have advice from someone whose situation and experience is more like your own than merely from the "authority." Much of inspiration for this book came from questions posted on the board, and I'm amazed at how new ones keep popping up. I hope you'll sign up and add some of your own.

Another thing people do at the bulletin board is report on their daily progress. There's a special "Daily Check-In" section of the site just for this. Some people check in semiformally using the Habit Traffic Light terminology I described in Chapter 6; others give a more free-form description of how they eat every day. Some people check in for just 21 days or for a calendar month, while they are building the habit; others have

been checking in for years. These check-ins are helpful both to the people who post them, because it gives
them a feeling of accountability, and to others who are
just browsing, because they can see that someone else
is actually doing this and can get a detailed, realistic
sense of what it takes.

Other things you'll see at the No S Diet bulletin
board are sporadic testimonials when some big mile-
stone has been reached ("My pants fell down!") and
cries for help in the event of some crisis ("It's two
hours till dinner and I'm hungry enough to eat a small
child, what should I do?"). It's a responsive, encour-
aging group, so requests for help tend to be promptly
answered, and milestones promptly congratulated.

The bulletin board is free. You don't even have to
register if all you want to do is browse existing messages. To post your own messages, you'll have to create an account, but that's free and easy, too. And don't
worry, I wouldn't in a million years think of spamming
you or selling your information to spammers. Don't be
shy about signing up. Internet bulletin boards can be
nasty, unforgiving places, but this board has an unusually kind and helpful membership. It's been a long time
since anyone has posted anything that could possibly
be interpreted as mean there.

HabitCal: An Online Habit Tracker

Using a paper calendar to track your behavior with
the Habit Traffic Light has some advantages: It's visually compelling to see these colored marks every day.
Reporting your progress on the Nosdiet.com bulletin

board has yet other advantages: You feel accountable to the group, part of a community. So I've created a third way that combines the strengths of both these methods of habit tracking: a free online habit calendar called the *HabitCal*. Conceptuallly, it works just like keeping a paper habit calendar, as I described in Chapter 6: You see an online calendar and mark off successful days in green, failures in red, and exempt S days in yellow.

I'm normally a big proponent of using the simplest possible technology to get the job done, but in this case I think the online calendar has an edge over paper. For one thing, paper calendars and markers might be cheap, but they do cost something. The online Habit-Cal is 100 percent free. This might not be much of a consideration if you're just tracking one habit, but if you're tracking multiple habits it can add up. The online HabitCal is also less labor-intensive to update; a single mouse click neatly fills in the whole box for each day, something that would be tedious to do by hand. You can see and edit data for multiple habits over multiple months on one screen. There is nothing to misplace. You can access it from anywhere.

But the greatest advantage may be the social aspect. When you keep your HabitCal online, you get the motivational benefit of knowing that other people (potentially at least) are keeping their eye on you. You have an audience for your struggles. You feel accountable to them. And if you run into trouble, it's a great diagnostic tool. Just invite other bulletin board members to take a look at your HabitCal and they can see at a glance how you've been doing instead of having to comb through hundreds of messages. They'll be able to quickly and accurately assess your situation and give you better advice.

The social aspect works two ways. As helpful as it is for others to be able to look at your HabitCal, you can learn a lot from looking at theirs, too. What level of compliance does it really take to see results on the No S Diet? Take a look at some successful No S Dieters' HabitCals, and you'll get a very precise idea of the range. Are there any other habits besides diet that it might make sense to track in this way? Get inspired by looking at what other people are doing.

You can find the HabitCal at www.everydaysystems .com/habitcal.

More Everyday Systems

Overeating wasn't the only bad habit I used to have. In fact, I had a whole litany: I drank too much alcohol, I smoked, I didn't exercise, I wasted a lot of time. But I was encouraged by my success in coming up with the No S Diet to take a crack at solving them, too; and some of the solutions I came up with also became quite successful—for me personally and for other people who read about them on my websites. Because these systems share conceptual underpinnings (S days, sustainable minimum of compliance, and so on) that seemed roughly analogous to computer software system components, I decided to call them *Everyday Systems*: mental software solutions for ordinary, everyday problems.

Though I haven't identified them as such, I've already mentioned a few of these Everyday Systems in passing throughout this book: Shovelglove (page 175), Urban Ranger (page 176), Glass Ceiling (page 54), and Intelligent Dietary Defaults (page 159). But there is a lot more to be said about each of them, and there are many more systems I haven't been able to touch on at all here. So if you have other bad habits besides overeating and are interested taking a No S–like approach to reforming them, take a look at the Everyday Systems hub site at www.everydaysystems.com.

What Next?

So you've made it to the end of this book. I'm impressed! Now what? What should you do *right now* to get started on this system?

Well, *start*. Don't give yourself a big, excessive last hurrah that is just going to leave you with a few more pounds to burn off—start now. You don't need any special equipment or food or training. You don't need to wait till any particular day of the week. You now know everything you need to know and have even heard most of it repeated several times. Just dive in.

Make a resolution to try the No S Diet *at least* through the next full calendar month. That should be enough time to build some real habit, provide a striking picture of your level of compliance if you are using the Habit Traffic Light, and give you a taste of what a

✳ The first month is as hard as it gets.

lifetime on the No S Diet would be like. And keep in mind that that first month is as hard as it gets. If you can make it past that, it's only going to get easier.

Scared you're not going to make it? That's okay. Most people slip up a few times before getting the habit firmly down. In fact, you should *expect* a few slipups. Use the Habit Traffic Light to feel in control even when your behavior hasn't been quite perfect, and remember that you can post to the free Nosdiet.com bulletin board if you are feeling discouraged or confused. But don't put off building strong new habits just because you know you have a lot of building left to do; that's all the more reason to start building now.

Best wishes, and looking forward to hearing lots of new No S Diet success stories,

—*Reinhard Engels and Ben Kallen*

Endnotes

Chapter 1

1. Centers for Disease Control and Prevention: National Center for Health Statistics, "Prevalence of Overweight and Obesity Among Adults: United States, 2003–2004." Available at www.cdc.gov/nchs/products/pubs/pubd/hestats/overweight/overwght_adult_03.htm. Accessed September 2007.

2. Business Wire, "Men's Fitness Announces the Current Crop of 'America's Fattest Cities 2003.'" Available at http://findarticles.com/p/articles/mi_m0ein/is_2003_jan_2/ai_96009094. Accessed September 2007.

3. Amber Waves: The Economics of Food, Farming, Natural Resources, and Rural America—U.S. Department of Agriculture, Economic Research Service, "U.S. Food Consumption Up 16 Percent Since 1970." Available at www.ers.usda.gov/amberwaves/november05/findings/usfoodconsumption.htm. Accessed September 2007.

4. Carol Krucoff, "When It Comes to Exercise, Little Things Mean a Lot," *Los Angeles Times*, March 25, 2002. Available at www.healingmoves.com/carol/articles/littlethings.html. Accessed September 2007.

5. Amber Waves: The Economics of Food, Farming, Natural Resources, and Rural America—U.S. Department of Agriculture, Economic Research Service, "U.S. Food Consumption Up 16 Percent Since 1970." Available at www

.ers.usda.gov/amberwaves/november05/findings/us
foodconsumption.htm. Accessed September 2007.

6. F. Bellisle, R. McDevitt, and A. M. Prentice, "Meal Frequency and Energy Balance," *British Journal of Nutrition* 77, Suppl. 1 (April 1997): S57–70. Available at www.ncbi
.nlm.nih.gov/sites/entrez?cmd=retrieve&db=pubmed&list
_uids=9155494&dopt=abstractplus. Accessed September
2007.

7. D. M. Cutler, E. L. Glaeser, and J. M. Shapiro. "Why Have Americans Become More Obese?" *Journal of Economic Perspectives* 17, no. 3 (Summer 2003): 93–118. Available at http://links.jstor.org/sici?sici=0895-3309(200
322)17%3A3%3C93%3AWHABMO%3E2.0.CO%3B2
-K. Accessed September 2007.

8. Science Daily, "Why Some People Get Fat and Others Don't: Too Much Snacking and Too Little Moving, Says Cornell Obesity Specialist." Available at www.sciencedaily
.com/releases/2000/02/000208075502.htm. Accessed September 2007.

9. L. Cordain, S. B. Eaton, A. Sebastian, et al. "Origins and Evolution of the Western Diet: Health Implications for the 21st Century," *American Journal of Clinical Nutrition* 81, no. 2 (February 2005): 341–354. Available at www.ajcn.org/
cgi/content/full/81/2/341. Accessed September 2007.

10. Brian Wansink, *Mindless Eating: Why We Eat More Than We Think* (New York: Bantam, 2006), 56.

11. U.S. Food and Drug Administration, "The Facts About Weight Loss Products and Programs." Available at http://
vm.cfsan.fda.gov/~dms/wgtloss.html. Accessed September
2007.

12. Michael Pollan, "Unhappy Meals," *The New York Times Magazine*, January 28, 2007. Available at www.nytimes
.com/2007/01/28/magazine/28nutritionism.t.html?ei=5088
&en=7c85a1c254546157&ex=1327640400&pagewanted
=all. Accessed September 2007.

Chapter 2

1. D. M. Cutler, E. L. Glaeser, and J. M. Shapiro. "Why Have Americans Become More Obese?" *Journal of Economic Perspectives* 17, no. 3 (Summer 2003): 101. Available at http://links.jstor.org/sici?sici=0895-3309(200322)17%3A 3%3C93%3AWHABMO%3E2.0.CO%3B2-K. Accessed September 2007.

2. Ibid.

3. L. S. Adair and B. M. Popkin, "Are Child Eating Patterns Being Transformed Globally?" *Obesity Research* 13, no. 7 (2005): 1281–1299.

4. WebMD, "The French feast on rich food, yet they remain slim. How do they do it?" Available at www.webmd .com/content/pages/10/1671_51408. Accessed September 2007.

5. Ibid.

6. Elisabeth Rosenthal, "Even the French are fighting obesity," *International Herald Tribune*, May 4, 2005. Available at www.iht.com/articles/2005/05/03/news/obese.php. Accessed September 2007.

7. Ibid.

8. C. E. Waller, S. Du, and B. M. Popkin, "Patterns of Overweight, Inactivity, and Snacking in Chinese Children," *Obesity Research* 11, no. 8 (2003): 957–961. Available at www .obesityresearch.org/cgi/content/full/11/8/957. Accessed September 2007.

9. L. Cleveland, J. Goldman, and A. Moshfegh, "Contribution of Snacks to Food and Nutrient Intakes in the United States," *The Federation of American Societies for Experimental Biology Journal* 19, no. 4 (2005): A88. Available at www.ars.usda.gov/research/publications/publications. htm?seq_no_115=171206. Accessed September 2007.

10. L. L. Hardy, L. A. Baur, S. P. Garnett, et al., "Family and Home Correlates of Television Viewing in 12–13 Year Old Adolescents: The Nepean Study," *International Journal of Behavioral Nutrition and Physical Activity* 29, no. 6 (2005): 711–719. Available at www.pubmedcentral.nih

.gov/articlerender.fcgi?artid=1594572. Accessed September 2007.

11. Ibid.

12. Jorge Cruise, *The 3-Hour Diet: How Low-Carb Diets Make You Fat and Timing Makes You Thin* (New York: HarperCollins, 2005).

13. H. Bertéus Forslund, J. S. Torgerson, L. Sjöström, et al., "Snacking Frequency in Relation to Energy Intake and Food Choices in Obese Men and Women Compared to a Reference Population," *International Journal of Obesity* 29 (2005): 711–719. Available at www.ncbi.nlm.nih.gov/sites/entrez?cmd=retrieve&db=pubmed&list_uids=15809664&dopt=abstractplus. Accessed September 2007.

14. A. Sanchez-Villegas, "Relative Role of Physical Inactivity and Snacking Between Meals in Weight Gain," *Medicina Clínica* 119, no. 2 (2002): 46–52

15. Craig Lambert, "The Way We Eat Now: Ancient Bodies Collide with Modern Technology to Produce a Flabby, Disease-Ridden Populace," *Harvard Magazine*, May–June 2004. Available at www.harvardmagazine.com/on-line/050465.html. Accessed September 2007.

16. American Dental Association, "Diet and Oral Health: Frequently Asked Questions." Available at www.ada.org/public/topics/diet_faq.asp. Accessed August 2007.

17. Leslie Pepper, "7 Secret Ways French Women Stay Slim," *Cosmopolitan*, February 2003. Available at www.lesliepepper.com/writer/detail.asp?content=5&category=2. Accessed September 2007.

18. D. M. Cutler, E. L. Glaeser, and J. M. Shapiro, "Why Have Americans Become More Obese?" *Journal of Economic Perspectives* 17, no. 3 (Summer 2003): 101. Available at http://links.jstor.org/sici?sici=0895-3309(200322)17%3A3%3C93%3AWHABMO%3E2.0.CO%3B2-K. Accessed September 2007.

19. Amber Waves: The Economics of Food, Farming, Natural Resources, and Rural America—U.S. Department of

Agriculture, Economic Research Service, "Trends in U.S. Per Capita Consumption of Dairy Products, 1909–2001." Available at www.ers.usda.gov/amberwaves/june03/pdf/awjune2003datafeature.pdf. Accessed September 2007.

20. "Why We're So Fat: Fast Food at School, Huge Portions, and Relentless TV Ads Make It Easy," *BusinessWeek*, October 21, 2002. Available at www.businessweek.com/magazine/content/02_42/b3804082.htm. Accessed September 2007.

21. Amber Waves: The Economics of Food, Farming, Natural Resources, and Rural America—U.S. Department of Agriculture, Economic Research Service, "U.S. Food Consumption Up 16 Percent Since 1970." Available at www.ers.usda.gov/amberwaves/november05/findings/usfoodconsumption.htm. Accessed September 2007.

Chapter 3

1. Amber Waves: The Economics of Food, Farming, Natural Resources, and Rural America—U.S. Department of Agriculture, Economic Research Service, "Estimating Consumption of Caloric Sweeteners." Available at www.ers.usda.gov/amberwaves/april03/indicators/behinddata.htm. Accessed September 2007.

2. Ibid.

3. L. Cordain, S. B. Eaton, A. Sebastian, et al. "Origins and Evolution of the Western Diet: Health Implications for the 21st Century," *American Journal of Clinical Nutrition* 81, no. 2 (February 2005): 341–354.

4. B. M. Popkin and S. J. Nielsen, "The Sweetening of the World's Diet," *Obesity Research* 11 (2003): 1325–1332.

5. Ice Cream USA, "Frequently Asked Questions." Available at http://icecreamusa.custhelp.com/cgi-bin/icecreamusa.cfg/php/enduser/std_adp.php?p_sid=2I6dvVKi&p_lva=&p_faqid=313&p_created=1124126438&p_sp=cF9zcmN oPTEmcF9ncmlkc29ydD0mcF9yb3dfY250PTEmcF 9zZWFyY2hfdGV4dD00NSBwaW50cyZwX3Byb2R

fbHZsMT1_YW55fiZwX2NhdF9sdmwxPX5hbnl_
JnBfcGFnZT0x&p_li=. Accessed September 2007.

6. Center for Science in the Public Interest, "Liquid Candy: How Soft Drinks Are Harming America's Health." Available at www.cspinet.org/liquidcandy. Accessed September 2007.

7. Ibid.

8. U.S. Office of the Surgeon General, Public Health Service, "The Surgeon General's Report on Nutrition and Health (1988)," 110. Available at http://profiles.nlm.nih.gov/NN/B/C/Q/N/_/nnbcqn.pdf. Accessed September 2007.

9. "Meat and the Planet," *International Herald Tribune*, December 27, 2006. Available at www.iht.com/articles/2006/12/27/opinion/edmeat.php. Accessed August 2007.

10. D. Grassi, C. Lippi, S. Necozione, et al., "Short-Term Administration of Dark Chocolate Is Followed by a Significant Increase in Insulin Sensitivity and a Decrease in Blood Pressure in Healthy Persons," *American Journal of Clinical Nutrition* 81, no. 3 (2005): 611–614. Available at www.ajcn.org/cgi/content/full/81/3/611. Accessed September 2007.

11. BBC News, "Chocolate 'Has Health Benefits': Eating Dark Chocolate Could Help Control Diabetes and Blood Pressure, Italian Experts Say," March 22, 2005. Available at http://news.bbc.co.uk/2/hi/health/4371867.stm. Accessed September 2007.

12. H. Schroeter, C. Heiss, J. Balzer, et al., "Epicatechin Mediates Beneficial Effects of Flavanol-Rich Cocoa on Vascular Function in Humans," *Proceedings of the National Academy of Sciences of the United States of America* 103, no. 4 (2006): 1024–1029. Available at www.pnas.org/cgi/content/full/103/4/1024. Accessed September 2007.

13. Center for Science in the Public Interest, "Liquid Candy: How Soft Drinks Are Harming America's Health." Available at www.cspinet.org/liquidcandy. Accessed September 2007.

Chapter 4

1. Brian Wansink, *Mindless Eating: Why We Eat More Than We Think* (New York: Bantam, 2006), 56.

2. Amber Waves: The Economics of Food, Farming, Natural Resources, and Rural America—U.S. Department of Agriculture, Economic Research Service, "U.S. Food Consumption Up 16 Percent Since 1970." Available at www.ers.usda.gov/amberwaves/november05/findings/usfood consumption.htm. Accessed September 2007.

Chapter 6

1. Sally Squires, "Week 1: Now, the Everyday Challenge," *The Washington Post*, January 8, 2002, HE01.

2. Nassim Nicholas Taleb, *Fooled by Randomness*, 2nd ed. (New York: Random House, 2005), 65.

3. Centers for Disease Control and Prevention, "Overweight and Obesity." Available at www.cdc.gov/nccdphp/dnpa/obesity. Accessed September 2007.

4. J. O. Hill and F. L. Trowbridge, "Childhood Obesity: Future Directions and Research Priorities," *Pediatrics* 101, no. 3 (1998, Suppl.): 571.

5. Craig Lambert, "The Way We Eat Now: Ancient Bodies Collide with Modern Technology to Produce a Flabby, Disease-Ridden Populace," *Harvard Magazine*, May–June 2004. Available at www.harvardmagazine.com/on-line/050465.html. Accessed September 2007.

6. U.S. Food and Drug Administration, "The Facts About Weight Loss Products and Programs." Available at http://vm.cfsan.fda.gov/~dms/wgtloss.html. Accessed September 2007.

Chapter 7

1. Michael Pollan, "Unhappy Meals," *The New York Times Magazine*, January 28, 2007. Available at www.nytimes

.com/2007/01/28/magazine/28nutritionism.t.html?ei=5088 &en=7c85a1c254546157&ex=1327640400&pagewanted =all. Accessed September 2007.

2. Brian Wansink, *Mindless Eating: Why We Eat More Than We Think* (New York: Bantam, 2006), 187.

About the Authors

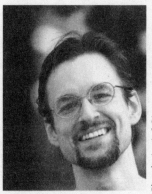

Reinhard Engels studied English literature and library science but somehow wound up as a software engineer at the Broad Institute of Harvard and MIT, where he develops genomic visualization tools. Despite the fact that he earns his bread and butter doing science, he doesn't think personal weight loss is a problem that requires deep scientific understanding. It certainly didn't in his case—he lost 40 pounds following the simple, commonsense rules described in this book and has kept them off for five years now. He lives with his wife and two daughters in Cambridge, Massachusetts.

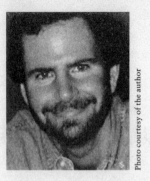

Ben Kallen has been writing about health and nutrition, as well as entertainment and the arts, for the past 15 years. His work has appeared in *Men's Fitness*, *Shape*, *Shape Cooks*, *Fit Pregnancy*, *Muscle & Fitness*, *Maximum Fitness*, *Natural Health*, *Body & Soul*, and WebMD.com, along with *Entertainment Weekly*, *TV Guide*, *Movieline*, *Los Angeles Magazine*, and the *Los Angeles Times*. He's been a staff writer and editor for *Men's Fitness* and *Shape*, among other publications, and was personal growth editor for Amazon.com. He lives in Santa Monica, California.